Shin So Shiatsu

Healing the Deeper Meridian Systems

Second Edition

Tetsuro Saito

Shin So Shiatsu – Healing the Deeper Meridian Systems
ISBN: 978-1-897435-74-8
Shin So Shiatsu – Practitioner's Reference Manual
ISBN: 978-1-897435-75-5

Copyright © 2006 Tetsuro Saito
Copyright © Second Edition 2012 Tetsuro Saito

All rights reserved.
No part of this publication may be reproduced, stored in a retrieval system, or transmitted in any form or by any means, electronic, mechanical, photocopying, recording or otherwise without the prior written permission of the author.

Note for librarians:
a cataloguing record to this book is available from Library and Archives Canada at
www.collectionscanada.ca/amicus/index-e.html

First Edition published as ISBN: 978-1-4251-0174-9

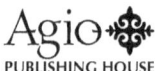

Agio Publishing House
151 Howe Street Victoria, BC   V8V 4K5 Canada
phone 250.380.0998
www.agiopublishing.com

More information: www.shinso-shiatsu.com

10 9 8 7 6 5 4 3 2 1

Shin So Shiatsu

Healing the Deeper Meridian Systems

Second Edition

Tetsuro Saito
Edited by Cheryl Coull

Credits

Editing: Cheryl Coull
Editorial assistance: Lesley Hamilton
Book design and layout: Rumiko Kanesaka
Computer support: Brian Smallshaw
Illustrations: Diana Lynn Thompson, Brian Smallshaw, Rumiko Kanesaka, Meriel Cammell, and Don Craig
Photography:
Shin So Shiatsu photos by Robin Grant and Juergen Raeuber
Scenic photos by Jean Belondrade (www.belondrade.com), Dorothy Haegert, Brian Smallshaw, and John Lutz
Calligraphy: Noriko Maeda
Cover photo and concept: Robin Grant
Cover design: Rumiko Kanesaka
Photo models: Cheryl Coull and Meriel Cammell
Assistance with editorial, design, and photography:
Peter Skrivanic, Meriel Cammell, Philippe Valerio, Rennard Lusterio, and Deidre Tessman

Acknowledgements

First and foremost, to my wife Kathi and my daughters Monika and Olivia, I would like to express my deepest gratitude. My greatest sacrifice through so many years of intensive research was time with my family. Without their understanding and support, this work would not exist.

Heartfelt thanks to:

- My shiatsu masters: Tokujiro Namikoshi, Toru Namikoshi, and Shizuto Masunaga. From them, I learned not only the skills and knowledge that come with formal shiatsu training, I learned about human nature. These great masters also helped build the very foundations of shiatsu in Canada.

- Tadashi Irie Sensei, who taught me the Finger Test Method upon which this entire body of meridian research has relied.

- My respected colleagues Hideo Yoshimoto M.D., Taku Yokoyama, and Yoshiko Sugioka who generously shared their valuable research with me.

- My longtime colleagues and friends, Pamela Ferguson (US), Akinobu Kishi (Japan), Norishiko Indei (US), Jean Lecomte (Canada), Tanya Harris (Canada), Lucie Poirier (Canada), Kazunobu Kamiya (Canada), Lawrence Hayword (Canada), Telse Hunter (US), Meredith S. Keator (US) as well as the members of the Shiatsu Centre and Shiatsu Research International.

- My European Shin So Shiatsu colleagues: Zita Sieber (Switzerland), Beatrix Simak (Austria), Peter Simak (Austria), Pietro Roat (Italy), and Matthias Wieck (Germany) whose concerted efforts have helped build a thriving European Shin So Shiatsu community.

- My Canadian Shin So Shiatsu colleagues: Lesley Hamilton, Heike Raschl, and Peter Skrivanic (Toronto, Canada); Cheryl Coull, Meriel Cammell, and Robin Grant (Victoria, Canada).

Finally, I must also acknowledge the ancient masters who developed the rich and fascinating system of Oriental medicine in which my work is rooted.

Foreword

A New World with Shin So Shiatsu
by Dr. Hideo Yoshimoto

Tetsuro Saito has written a tremendously significant book, one with the potential to overturn centuries of "common sense" in Eastern medicine.

Written for the purpose of training shiatsu therapy graduates, it is the fruit of Mr. Saito's sincere life-long work as a shiatsu therapist and researcher. The result is astonishing and will change many of Eastern medicine's fixed concepts. For instance, the Saito Meridian Charts show the Large Intestine Meridian not only on the arms, but also on the legs. Therefore, if the patient's problem is deep, it could reach to the bottom of the foot, namely to Yusen (KD 1).

I was amazed when I first looked at the Saito Charts. I found it hard to believe that the Large Intestine Meridian extended to the legs. But by using the Finger Test Method, I realized this to be true. The Saito Charts have opened up a whole new world for me, and improved the results of my treatments.

By touching patients' bodies and through his never-ending research, Mr. Saito has developed and refined his sensitivity. While reading this book, I realized with astonishment that his Eastern medical experience had reached a depth far beyond that of acupuncture and moxabustion practitioners such as myself.

I first met and became good friends with Tetsuro through our mutual interest in the Finger Test Method, and it is such a pleasure to know he has accumulated the results of his research on this subject and made it available to us. This book offers all practitioners of Eastern medicine a new goal: that of attaining better results, and indeed, of devising a whole new way of practicing acupuncture and moxabustion based on the Saito Charts.

Just as Mr. Saito has gone beyond Zen Shiatsu, I sincerely hope this book can lead readers to a deeper realization of shiatsu and Eastern Medicine in general. May it help us all to become bright beacons for those who are suffering.

Hideo Yoshimoto, M.D., is highly regarded for his published research in both Eastern and Western medical approaches. He is a surgeon, acupuncturist, and medical herbalist. A prominent member of the Irie Finger Test Group, he lives in Saga Prefecture, Japan.

Foreword

Shiatsu — A Higher Form of Communication
by Akinobu Kishi

I first met Tetsuro Saito at the inaugural Meridian Shiatsu Conference in Berlin in the year 2000. Although we both graduated from the Nippon Shiatsu School (I in 1971, Mr. Saito three years earlier) we had never met before.

We had also both been members of Shizuto Masunaga's Iokai Institute — Mr. Saito while living in Canada, and myself in Europe — and had devoted much energy to study and practice since the early 1970s. During this time, Mr. Saito was also busy promoting shiatsu in his adopted home through many activities, including hosting several visits by Masunaga Sensei.

Though our paths had never crossed in the 30 years since our graduation, our first encounter was a truly enjoyable event. I felt like I was meeting an old friend.

Our friendship has deepened since then, at shiatsu conferences in Italy and Austria where we were both honoured as senior Japanese instructors, and in Canada where I have been privileged to conduct workshops as Mr. Saito's guest.

The Japanese art of shiatsu is well known nowadays, with conferences around the world facilitated by a new generation of non-Japanese practitioners. I am deeply moved when I reflect on how far our field has come, and how Japanese therapists like ourselves are being called upon to share our knowledge.

My deepest respect goes to Tetsuro Saito, who has worked with continuous and sincere devotion to develop and teach his Shin So Shiatsu system in the West, where the challenges of studying and practicing shiatsu can be monumental.

Shiatsu therapists today must develop not only a great depth of skill but also their own individual approaches. The Seiki-Soho system, which I have taught since 1980, and Tetsuro Saito's Shin So Shiatsu system are both responses to this demand.

But there is more. To bring ki into balance is to realize the unity of body and mind. It is also to understand the body's energetic flows and guide them into harmony with the flow from the Source. This is only possible through polishing our sensitivity of mind and body, which is, I believe, the true goal of shiatsu training.

I also believe that giving and receiving a shiatsu treatment is a higher form of communication. I look forward to the day when shiatsu therapy is understood as more than the integration of sensation, technique, and knowledge, and is embraced as a whole new field, in which we explore each other's resonance.

With this hope, I offer my words in support of Tetsuro Saito and his new book.

Kyoto, Japan
Early spring 2006,
the air fragrant with plum blossoms,
Akinobu Kishi

After graduating from the Japan Shiatsu School in 1971, Akinobu Kishi became Shizuto Masunaga's assistant. With roots in shiatsu, Shintoism, and traditional Japanese arts, he has developed his own Seiki-Soho approach and works with students from around the world.

Contents

• indicates instructions

Credits and Acknowledgements	iv
Foreword by Dr. Hideo Yoshimoto	vi
Foreword by Akinobu Kishi	vii
Contents	ix
Figures and Illustrations	xiii

Introduction — 1

Shin So Shiatsu: An Ancient Path to New Frontiers	1
What is Shin So Shiatsu?	3
How Does Shin So Shiatsu Work?	4
Why Practice Shin So Shiatsu?	5
What is in this Book?	7
How Does One Learn Shin So Shiatsu?	8
The Future of Shiatsu Therapy	8

Chapter 1 The Regular Meridians Revisited — 11

The TCM Acupuncture Chart: An Efficient Shorthand	14
The Twelve Meridians: Three Levels of Imbalance	15
What the Classics Say	16
Toward a More Complete Picture	16
Shizuto Masunaga: A Great Leap Forward	17
Beyond Zen Shiatsu: Saito Regular Meridians	20
Regular Meridians Up Close	22
An Overview of TCM Simplifications	24
Where They Flow	25
The Regular Meridians in General	25
Yin Regular Meridians in First and Second Degree	25
Yang Regular Meridians in First and Second Degree	26
Yin Regular Meridians in Third Degree	26
Yang Regular Meridians in Third Degree	28

Chapter 2 New Phenomena: Energy Circles and Meridian Belt Zones — 31

Meridian Diagnostic Zones are Energy Circles	34
Types of Energy Circles	36
Characteristics of Energy Circles	36
Meridian Belt Zones	37
Characteristics of Meridian Belt Zones	37
Comparing the Masunaga and Saito Back Charts	41
The Link Between Meridian Belt Zones and Meridian Stretch Positions	41
The Link Between Meridian Belt Zones and Organ Functions	42
The Hirata Zones	43

Chapter 3 Sensing Energy — 45

Listen with your Tanden — 47
Dr. Tadashi Irie: Inventor of the Finger Test Method — 48
Performing the Finger Test — 49
What are You Looking For? — 49
How the Finger Test Method Works — 49
Our Hands are Sensors — 49
• Preparing to perform the finger test — 50
• Performing the finger test — 51
Finger Testing Foods and Supplements — 52
• Finger testing foods and supplements — 52
Now Add Sound Imaging — 52
Dealing with Surface Ja ki — 53
Finger Test-imonials — 53
• Clearing surface ja ki — 54
More Practice with Sound Images — 56
• Locating a vertebra with sound imaging — 56
Sensing Meridians — 56
• Sensing Regular Meridians — 57
Sensing Abdominal Diagnostic Zones — 58
• Sensing abdominal diagnostic zones — 58

Chapter 4 Goals and Methods of Shin So Shiatsu — 59

About Sei Ki and Ja Ki — 61
How Internal Ja Ki is Created — 62
The Three Main Goals of Shin So Shiatsu — 63
The Two Main Components of a Shin So Treatment — 63
The Four Main Shin So Shiatsu Treatment Methods — 64
Diagnosing the Deepest Level of Imbalance — 65
• Diagnosing the deepest level of imbalance — 65
Determining a Focus: Structural or Internal — 65
• Determining a structural or internal treatment focus — 65
Locating Specific Structural Problems — 66
• Locating specific structural problems — 66
Shin So Shiatsu and Diode Treatment — 66
Treatment Responses — 67
• Using diodes with Shin So Shiatsu — 67
• Sealing off a ja ki source in a room — 67

Chapter 5 Diagnosing and Treating the Regular Meridians — 69

Regular Meridians in First Degree — 71
Regular Meridians in Second Degree — 71
Regular Meridians in Third Degree — 72
Four Key Meridians — 72
Diagnosing the Regular Meridians: Kyo and Jitsu — 73

- Diagnosing kyo and jitsu — 73
Confirming our Shin So Diagnosis — 73
- Confirming a kyo-jitsu diagnosis — 74
- Diagnosing which third-degree meridians need treatment — 74
- Diagnosing the most imbalanced second-degree meridians — 74
- Confirming your diagnosis of a third-degree yin meridian — 75
- Confirming your diagnosis of a third-degree yang meridian — 75
Magnetic Polarity of the Sensor — 76
Treating the Regular Meridians — 76
Belt Zones and Stretch Positions — 77
- Positioning the arm for Regular Meridian treatment — 78
- Positioning the leg for Regular Meridian treatment — 78
- Confirming correct leg and arm positioning — 79
The Importance of Treating Meridians on the Arms and Legs — 80
- Treating the most kyo and jitsu meridians on the arm and leg — 80
- Yin/yang Regular Meridian treatment on the arm — 80
- Yin/yang Regular Meridian treatment on the leg — 80
Shin So Shiatsu Master Points — 81

Chapter 6 Diagnosing and Treating the Extra Meridians — 83

The TCM View — 86
Toward a More Complete Picture — 87
A Note on Extra Meridian Names — 88
Hatsu-so-ketsu: Confluent Points — 89
Where They Flow: The Extra Meridians — 89
Links between the Regular and Extra Meridians — 90
Extra Meridian Energy Circles — 92
Extra Meridian Belt Zones — 94
Sensing the Extra Meridians — 94
- Sensing the Extra Meridians — 95
- Sensing Extra Meridian belt zones — 95
- Diagnosing the Extra Meridians — 96
Treating the Extra Meridians — 98
- Energy Circles and the yaki hari technique — 99
- Diagnosing Extra Meridian energy circles — 99
- Treating Extra Meridian energy circles with yaki hari — 100
- Treating localized structural problems with yaki hari — 101
- Diagnosing and treating pelvic imbalances — 102
- Treating Extra Meridians with shiatsu — 102
- Treating Extra Meridians by removing ja ki — 104
- Treating Extra Meridian Confluent Points with ion pumping cords — 106
- How to locate an acupuncture point — 107

Chapter 7 Diagnosing and Treating the Divergent Meridians — 109

The TCM View — 112
Toward a More Complete Picture — 113

Where They Flow: The Divergent Meridians	114
Crossing Points and Ratsu-ketsu Points	116
Diagnosing the Divergent Meridians	116
• Diagnosing the Divergent Meridians	117
Treating the Divergent Meridians	118
• Treating the Divergent Meridians with the yaki hari technique	118
• Treating the Divergent Meridians with shiatsu	120
• Treating the Divergent Meridians by removing ja ki	121
• Treating Divergent Meridians with IP cords	122
Treatment Summary	126

Chapter 8 Diagnosing and Treating the Oceans System — 127

The TCM View	129
Doctors Oda and Yoshimoto: Oceans System Pioneers	130
Toward a More Complete Picture	130
The Saito Ocean Zones	132
Where They Flow: The Oceans Meridians	133
Meridian Fundamentals	133
The Ocean Meridians	135
• Diagnosing imbalances in the Oceans System	136
Treating the Oceans System	137
• Treating the Oceans System with two-point ja ki removal	137
• Treating the Oceans System with Mu Bun Sai ja ki removal	138
• Detecting early imbalances in the Ocean Meridians	138

Chapter 9 Diagnosing and Treating the Tai Kyoku System — 139

Where they flow: Tai Kyoku Meridians	142
Diagnosing the Tai Kyoku System	144
• Diagnosing Tai Kyoku 1	144
• Diagnosing Tai Kyoku 2	144
Treating the Tai Kyoku System	145
• Treating the Tai Kyoku system by removing ja ki	145

Chapter 10 Diagnosing and Treating the Chakra System — 147

Toward a More Complete Picture	150
• Diagnosing chakras	151
• Treating chakras	151

In Conclusion — 153

Epilogue: Celebrating Milestones	154
About Tetsuro Saito	155
Shin So Shiatsu Studies	156
Suggested Reading	158
Index	160

Figures and Illustrations

The Regular Meridians Revisited

1-1 Spleen Meridian illustrated by Katsupaku Jin	14
1-2 Three levels of Regular Meridian imbalance	15
1-3 Shizuto Masunaga in Canada	17
1-4a Masunaga meridian chart	19
1-4b Abbreviation of meridian names	19
1-5a Masunaga's Large Intestine Meridian	20
1-5b-e Saito Large Intestine Meridian	21
1-6a A Regular Meridian: three lines of energy	22
1-6b Meridian energy: high and low density areas	22
1-7 Stomach Meridian	22
1-8 Acupuncture points on a meridian	22
1-9 Acupuncture points on a meridian	22
1-10 Acupuncture points on a meridian	23
1-11 A TCM meridian	23
1-12 Four TCM meridians	23
1-13a TCM Kidney Meridian	23
1-13b Saito Kidney Meridian	23
1-14 TCM and Saito Gallbladder meridians	24
1-15 TCM and Saito Small Intestine meridians	25
1-16 TCM and Saito Stomach meridians	25
1-17 Yin Regular Meridians: first and second degree	26
1-18 Yang Regular Meridians: first and second degree	26
1-19 Yin Regular Meridians in third degree	27
1-20 Yang Regular Meridians in third degree	28

New Phenomena: Energy Circles and Meridian Belt Zones

2-1 Masunaga's hara diagnostic chart	34
2-2a-c Saito Abdominal Diagnostic Charts: three levels	35
2-3a Saito Kidney Meridian zone	35
2-3b Saito Bladder Meridian zone	35
2-3c Masunaga's Bladder and Kidney zones	35
2-4a Spleen Meridian zone before treatment	37
2-4b Spleen Meridian zone after treatment	37
2-5 The Hirata Zones	38
2-6a-b Small Intestine belt zone: normal	39
2-7a-b Small Intestine belt zone: imbalanced	39
2-8a-g Regular Meridian belt zones in first degree	40
2-9a Masunaga's back diagnostic chart	41
2-9b Saito back diagnostic chart	41
2-10a Regular Meridian belt zones	41
2-10b Liver Meridian stretch positions	41
2-11 Belt zones occur in pairs	42
2-12 Belt zones mirror the body	42
2-13 Divergent Meridian belt zones	44

Sensing Energy

3-1 Dr. Tadashi Irie	48
3-2 The finger test works like a TV set	49
3-3 Our hands are extremely sensitive	50
3-4 How to finger test	51
3-5 Finger testing cigarettes	51
3-6 Ja ki covers us from the feet upwards	54
3-7a-f Clearing surface ja ki	55
3-8a First-degree sensor	56
3-8b Second-degree sensor	56
3-8c Third-degree sensor	56
3-9 General sensor	57
3-10 Sensing meridians using a chopstick	57
3-11 Sensing meridians using a chopstick	57
3-12 Stomach Meridian diagnostic zones	58
3-13 Approach energy circles from the outside in	58
3-14 Tracing a first-degree diagnostic zone	58

Goals and Methods of Shin So Shiatsu

4-1 Ja ki accumulates like sediment on a riverbottom	63
4-2 A diode	67

Diagnosing and Treating the Regular Meridians

5-1 Relationship between meridian imbalances and symptoms	72
5-2 Diagnosing kyo and jitsu	73
5-3 Using aluminum foil to confirm kyo-jitsu diagnosis	74

5-4 Finger testing the abdomen: third-degree sensor   74
5-5 Finger testing the abdomen: second-degree sensor   74
5-6 Confirmation points for yin meridians in third degree   75
5-7 Confirmation points for yang meridians in third degree   75
5-8 Confirming Bladder Meridian diagnosis   75
5-9a Regular Meridian Belt Zones   77
5-9b Stretch position for the Liver Meridian   77
5-10 Positioning leg for treatment of third-degree meridians   78
5-11 Arm positions for treatment   79
5-12 Shin So Master Points: neck and shoulder   81
5-13 Shin So Master Points: sacrum   81
5-14 Shin So Master Points: back of legs   81

Diagnosing and Treating the Extra Meridians

6-1 The Extra Meridians   86
6-2 Extra Meridian Confluent Points   87
6-3 TCM Extra Meridians   87
6-4 Jitsu energy flows into the Extra Meridians   88
6-5 Direction of Extra Meridian flow   89
6-6 Extra Meridians and structural integrity   90
6-7 Regular Meridians and the Extra Meridians they flow into   90
6-8 Yin and Yang Connecting Extra Meridians   91
6-9 Yang Connecting Meridian (wide band)   91
6-10 Yin Connecting Meridian (wide band)   91
6-11 Conception Meridian: face and feet   91
6-12 Extra Meridian energy circle locations   92
6-13 Energy Circles and associated Extra Meridians   92
6-14 Close-up view of Extra Meridian energy circles   93
6-15 Extra Meridian belt zones   94
6-16a Extra Meridian sound images   94
6-16b Extra Meridian sensor   94
6-17 Comparing Extra and Regular meridians   95
6-18 Sensing an Extra Meridian belt zone   95
6-19 Extra Meridian confirmation points   96
6-20 Energy circles on the abdomen   96
6-21 Yin and yang Extra Meridian flow on the leg   97
6-22 Yaki hari materials   99
6-23 An energy circle   100
6-24 Placing press needles in an energy circle   101
6-25 Energy circles reflect pelvic imbalance   102
6-26 Pelvis after yaki hari treatment   102
6-27a-b Leg positions for Extra Meridian treatment   103
6-28 Arm positions for Extra Meridian treatment   103
6-29a-b Mu Bun Sai Ja Ki charts   104
6-30 Shin So Shiatsu Ja Ki Chart   104
6-31 Mu Bun Sai chart showing ja ki   104
6-32 IP cord connecting Confluent Points   106
6-33 Confluent Points for Extra Meridian IP-cord treatment   107

Diagnosing and Treating the Divergent Meridians

7-1 Divergent Meridians and associated organs   112
7-2 Dr. Irie's Divergent Meridian charts   113
7-3a Lung Divergent Meridian   114
7-3b Large Intestine Divergent Meridian   114
7-4 Large Intestine Divergent Meridian flow on feet   114
7-5 Lung and Spleen Divergent Meridians: arms and legs   114
7-6 Divergent Meridian flow along spine   115
7-7 Flow pattern for imbalanced yang Divergent Meridians   115
7-8 Flow pattern for imbalanced yin Divergent Meridians   116
7-9 Intersection points for Divergent Meridians   116
7-10 Ratsu-ketsu Points   116
7-11 Divergent Meridian sensor   117
7-12 Confirmation points for Divergent Meridian imbalances   117
7-13 Divergent Meridian flow to Heart   119
7-14 Divergent Meridian confirmation point   119
7-15 Positioning leg for Divergent Meridian treatment   121
7-16 Arm positions for Divergent Meridian treatment   121
7-17a-b Divergent Meridian Crossing Points on upper body   123
7-18a-b Ratsu-ketsu Points on arms   123
7-19a-b Ratsu-ketsu Points on legs   123
7-20 IP-cord sequence for Lung Divergent Meridian   124
7-21 IP-cord sequence for Gallbladder Divergent Meridian   124
7-22 Divergent treatment: secondary meridians   124
7-23 Two-cord sequence: Lung Divergent Meridian   125
7-24 Two-cord sequence: Gallbladder Divergent Meridian   125

Diagnosing and Treating the Oceans System

8-1 Oceans Regulating Points identified by TCM	129
8-2 Dr. Oda's sound images for the six Oceans	130
8-3 Two branches of energy flow into the Oceans	131
8-4 From sea to sky: the Oceans System	132
8-5 Regular Meridian flow into the Oceans	132
8-6 Extra Meridian flow into the Oceans	132
8-7 Meridians and their functions	134
8-8 Ki Kai zone and Spleen Ocean Meridian	135
8-9 Saito Ocean Zones	136
8-10 Oceans sensor	136
8-11 Saito Oceans System confirmation points	136
8-12 Oceans treatment leg positions	137
8-13 Ocean zones, sounds, and associated meridians	137
8-14 Arm positions for Oceans treatment	137

Diagnosing and Treating the Tai Kyoku System

9-1 Tai Kyoku 1 meridians	142
9-2 Tai Kyoku 2 meridians	142
9-3 Tai Kyoku 1 energy circle	142
9-4 Tai Kyoku 2 energy circle	142
9-5 Tai Kyoku 1 meridian and treatment points	143
9-6 Tai Kyoku 1: six yang energy pathways	143
9-7 Tai Kyoku 2 meridian and treatment points	143
9-8 Tai Kyoku 2: six yin energy pathways	143
9-9 Tai Kyoku 1 sensor	144
9-10 Tai Kyoku 1 confirmation point	144
9-11 Tai Kyoku 2 sensor	145
9-12 Tai Kyoku 2 confirmation point	145

Diagnosing and Treating the Chakra System

10-1 Yoshimoto Chakra Sensor	149
10-2 Major and minor chakras	149
10-3 Chakra Meridians front view	150
10-4 Chakra Meridians back view	150
10-5 Chakras and their links with the organs	150
10-6 The 6th Chakra governs the ears and eyes	150
10-7 Treating Chakras	151

Introduction

Shin So Shiatsu
An Ancient Path to New Frontiers

Oriental medicine is one of the world's oldest and most widely known medical systems, despite having been acknowledged in the West for less than five decades. Its foundation, the meridian system, observed and studied for at least 2,000 years, has the potential to become one of the future's most promising avenues of healing.

What we know of Oriental medicine today, however, is only a fraction of what was once understood. Much has been lost to the tides of history and we have been left with only a basic working knowledge of the ancient and complex diagnostic system we now refer to as Traditional Chinese Medicine (TCM). TCM is nonetheless a profoundly effective system, rich in clues that can help us recover much of what has been forgotten or omitted, and in clues that can guide us toward completely new discoveries.

The main obstacle in advancing our knowledge of the body's energy matrix is that few practitioners innately possess the sensitivity required to accurately and confidently sense the flow of energy, or ki, within the human body.

It is to this task that I have devoted my life as a therapist and researcher: to finding and developing an approach that enables dedicated practitioners to perceive and work precisely with meridian flow.

At the heart of this book is the Finger Test Method, which has given me, and a growing community of others, the ability to read the body's energetic patterns. The story of how I came upon this simple technique, the discoveries it has led me to, and its evolution into the system of diagnosis and treatment I call Shin So, or "deeper level" Shiatsu, unfolds in the chapters to follow.

This is more than a story about my research. It's the story about the path I stepped onto, and the many teachers, researchers, and practitioners whose own lifelong quests built that path. The greatest gift is the gift of knowledge. My deepest gratitude goes to the sages whose classical writings we are still exploring, to Shizuto Masunaga and Tokujiru Namikoshi, the fathers of shiatsu as we know it today. And to the acupuncturist Dr. Tadashi Irie who developed the Finger Test Method and generously shared it with me, and supported me in my research.

It was thanks to Dr. Irie's pioneering work that I began the task of tracing and mapping the flow of the 12 Regular Meridians. As I became more adept with the technique, I went on to uncover the complex interrelationships between these "main" meridians and the deeper Extra, Divergent, Ocean, and Cosmic systems.

Over the years, this work has proven both challenging and exhilarating. I have often felt as if I was on a jungle expedition in search of hidden treasure. Many times, I have been lost and forced back to the starting point. Many times, I have experienced the elation of uncovering something completely new and potentially very useful, only to learn my "discovery" had already been chronicled by the ancient masters. At other times, I have been most fortunate that invaluable insights and guidance have come to me via my dreams.

The greatest highlights of this undulating journey have been in bringing new approaches to my patients. The joy I feel in finding ways to help them is more than enough to make me forget wrong turns and relentless searching. Yet even here, there have been failures and disappointments. I have come to appreciate this as the nature of research.

I have used the Finger Test Method faithfully in my own practice for nearly two decades now, and it continues to refine and expand my meridian research. It has proven invaluable, reliable, and, perhaps most importantly, transmissible. Many of my students throughout North America and Europe, shiatsu practitioners for many years, had given up on ever being able to locate meridians precisely, relying on charts and some degree of intuition. But after attending just their first Shin So Shiatsu workshop, they were very excited to find themselves accurately tracing these pathways.

While I have written this book primarily for shiatsu therapists, acupuncturists and other practitioners with a basic theoretical and working background in meridian therapy, it is my wish that it offer insight and inspiration to anyone drawn to working with the meridians as a diagnostic and treatment tool. Newcomers to the field will find it useful to explore existing works introducing shiatsu, which are cited in the bibliography at the end of the book.

What is Shin So Shiatsu?

Shin So Shiatsu enables any practitioner to sense and precisely trace the multitude of meridian pathways in the human body, to identify the levels at which energy imbalances occur, and treat those imbalances. We don't memorize where meridians and treatment points are; we feel where they are.

Shin So Shiatsu is what shiatsu becomes when we are able to sense energy and work with it in very precise ways. It is what evolved naturally from my three decades of research and practice with Masunaga's legacy, Dr. Irie's Finger Test Method, and a system of sound diagnosis all incorporated into a detailed, practical, and accurate method of diagnosing and treating patients.

Shin So Shiatsu (深層指圧) translates directly into English as "deeper level shiatsu." On a most literal level, this refers to its embrace of the deeper levels of the energy matrix. In other words, Shin So Shiatsu addresses not only the 12 Regular Meridians that most meridian-based shiatsu styles focus on, it also actively engages the less-known, extremely important Extra, Divergent, Ocean, and Cosmic meridian systems.

More than this, Shin So adds a deeper level to our personal exploration of shiatsu. It urges us to work from our tandens and our spirits. It gives our practices, and our lives, a sense of purpose and progress. It brings to our workday the excitement of being on an adventure; the feeling that, finally, we're on to something — that same "something" that drew us to shiatsu in the first place.

How Does Shin So Shiatsu Work?

We can see the interplay of energy systems within the human body as a microcosm of the world around us (this is illustrated in figure 8-4 on page 132).

Rain falls to Earth, filling intricate networks of rivers and streams. These waterways flow through vast and varied terrains to reach, as their final destination, the ocean. Immeasurable volumes of water flow seaward continuously, and yet, thanks to the powerful energy of the sun and the process of evaporation, we are not inundated. This evaporation creates more clouds and more rain, which again, falls to Earth.

This cycle repeats itself within the human body. Our bodies are like the Earth. The energy that fills the cosmos and is absorbed into us is like the rain. This cosmic energy accumulates and flows throughout our bodies via the Regular Meridian system. From time to time, in order to regulate the energy volume, major tributaries — the Extra and Divergent Meridians — will siphon off some of this ocean-bound flow. The flow finally enters the Oceans System, and from there is re-absorbed into the Tai Kyoku (Cosmic) System. Meanwhile, our bodies absorb fresh Cosmic Energy.

Such adjustments in energy levels are very specific responses to the body's needs. Disturbances from either within our bodies, or without, will elicit a cascade of reactions — engaging first the Regular Meridians, then the Extra Meridians, and, when the disturbance is strong enough or persistent enough, the Divergent Meridians, and even the Ocean and Cosmic energy systems.

In striving to regain homeostasis and reduce the strain being placed upon it, this complicated multi-meridians system will "ask" for assistance. This is where Shin So Shiatsu enters the scene. Our approach is to identify the deepest level at which this effort is taking place, eliminate the disturbance, support the meridian system in question, and restore balance to it.

Our diagnosis of a patient may reveal, for example, that only their Regular Meridian system is engaged in such a regulatory response. We say, in other words, the Regular Meridian system is "out of balance." We may proceed to find that this imbalance has engaged the Regular

Meridians as they manifest in their third degree, i.e. the deepest level within this system. We identify precisely which of these third-degree meridians are most affected: which one is the most kyo and which one is the most jitsu. By treating and re-balancing just these two meridians, the remaining 10 will also fall into balance. We do not need to treat all 12 Regular Meridians one by one.

In another situation, we may find that body's effort to fend off dis-ease has penetrated beyond the Regular Meridians to affect the Extra and Divergent Meridian systems. What do we do?

We treat the Divergent Meridians first. And remarkably, in doing this, balance will be restored to both the Extra and Regular Meridian systems even though they do not directly receive treatment.

In this case, if we were to address only the Regular Meridians and not the Divergent Meridians, we might be able to achieve balance — but only in the Regular Meridians. And the dis-ease, still rooted in the deeper system, would quickly push the Regular Meridian system out of balance again. Although we might see an improvement in the patient's condition, it would only be temporary, and the individual would soon be seeking help again.

Practitioners of Shizuto Masunaga's Zen Shiatsu approach have been trained to work only with the Regular Meridians. I have come to realize this is not enough: in addressing the deeper meridian systems, our treatments will be more effective than we could ever imagine. Masunaga Sensei devoted his life to building the foundations of meridian shiatsu. To honour his efforts, it is time to take his work this step further.

Why Practice Shin So Shiatsu?

Shiatsu therapists have traditionally relied on touch — palpation of the hara or back — to diagnose meridian imbalances. Shin So Shiatsu uses the Finger Test Method to obtain very specific information from a vast array of reflex zones and meridians throughout the body.

There are important advantages to using this method. Firstly, diagnostic speed and accuracy can be quickly achieved. Years of special training are needed to master the more traditional palpation skills, and few ever attain a level that will make this a reliable method for them. Working with the finger test actually facilitates development of better palpation skills.

Secondly, the Shin So approach has a built-in system for confirming diagnoses. This has been a huge challenge with the palpation method, where practitioners, unless gifted with exceptional sensitivity, are rarely able to corroborate one another's results. I have seen many therapists lose confidence and eventually abandon diagnosis altogether because of this uncertainty. Confirmation helps clarify and strengthen our treatments.

Thirdly, the finger test allows Shin So Shiatsu therapists to pinpoint structural and alignment problems, locate the source of joint or muscle pain, and diagnose other conditions.

Fourthly, in the very dynamic ki-meridian system, we can feel fluctuations as they occur. We can feel pathways becoming more or less unbalanced. At the end of a Shin So treatment, we will know whether the patient's meridian system has been balanced or still needs work.

The finger test is a powerful tool for diagnosing, confirming and reassessing imbalances, but even more importantly, it increases the depth and manner of our communication with the ki-meridian system, giving us direct access to energy dimensions that until now have been out of our reach.

Other Benefits of the Shin So Shiatsu System

- The key elements of Shin So Shiatsu can be integrated into any shiatsu style, as well as acupuncture and other forms of therapy. I consider shiatsu an art: each therapist is an individual, each treatment unique. Shin So Shiatsu encourages and facilitates this.

- The practice of Shin So Shiatsu cultivates in us a greater sense of presence and self awareness and helps bring our own energy into better balance. Our treatments become more efficient, less labour intensive. After a day of Shin So treatments, we feel refreshed and inspired.

- Shin So Shiatsu can be integrated into our daily lives. With the finger test, we can test our own and our children's energetic receptivity to certain foods; we can determine how close we can sit to the television or computer before we begin to absorb too much surface ja ki. In the event that we do absorb it, we can also clear it away.

- The community of Shin So practitioners is growing worldwide. For information sharing and training opportunities, see page 156.

What is in this Book?

This book contains the theoretical and practical information you will need to become proficient in the art of Shin So Shiatsu. Carry it with you everywhere: to your Shin So Shiatsu workshops, your treatment space, the summer cottage, and breakfast table.

In Chapter 1 you will find a review of the Regular Meridian system with which you are likely most familiar. You will see in plain terms how this seemingly one-dimensional grid, as presented on contemporary TCM charts, has its own "deeper levels."

This more detailed view of the Regular Meridians is part of that ancient body of Oriental medical theory lost to us for a time. This recovered knowledge provides a context for exciting new findings, such as those described in Chapter 2, linking meridians to energy circles and meridian belt zones.

Chapter 3 puts you in the driver's seat with specific instructions for performing the Finger Test Method and sound imaging. You will practice tracing meridians, energy circles, and meridian belt zones. Chapter 4 provides you with some general rules of the road — basic principles of Shin So Shiatsu — before you receive detailed instructions for the Shin So diagnosis and treatment of the Regular, Extra, Divergent, Ocean, and Tai Kyoku (Cosmic) systems in Chapters 5, 6, 7, 8, 9, and 10.

All of this is accompanied by the *Shin So Shiatsu Practitioner's Reference Manual*, which contains your navigational aids: the finger test sensors, meridian charts, and sound images that you will need to practice Shin So Shiatsu. While you will find it helpful to gradually memorize the sensors and sound images, the meridian charts are there simply to reassure you that you are on track. There is no other way to learn than by doing. Don't hesitate to flip the *Reference Manual* open and refer to it during a treatment: your patients won't mind.

How Does One Learn Shin So Shiatsu?

The basic techniques of Shin So Shiatsu can be learned quickly, and as soon as you are introduced to them you will be able to feel meridian energy. While learning the system, students benefit profoundly by being able to "tune in" to the energy of an experienced teacher. The teacher also helps them interpret what they are feeling on an energetic level.

Shin So Shiatsu is taught as a post-graduate course for shiatsu practitioners (or when appropriate, those experienced in other forms of bodywork or energy work). It is usually offered in a series of five or more intensive three- or four-day workshops each scheduled five to six months apart. Between workshops, review days help keep students in tune with their new practice. For more information, see page 156.

The Future of Shiatsu Therapy

The three decades of research described in this book have opened up new avenues for diagnosis and treatment. Major outcomes include:

- A complete charting of the flow patterns for the Regular, Extra, and Divergent meridians, and thorough descriptions of the Ocean and Cosmic energy systems;

- A more complete understanding of the relationships between each of these systems and the development of methods to determine just when, where, and how, one system engages with another;

- New charts to facilitate diagnosis and treatment;

- The development of new treatment protocols for each system.

It is my hope that these developments will offer therapists better tools to help their patients deal with more serious levels of imbalance, as well as encourage and inspire others to carry out more research in this field. For many years, members of our profession have struggled to understand more deeply the implications of energetic imbalances in the body. I believe that through this research we can accomplish this and develop even more effective, more powerful treatments.

1
Regular Meridians Revisited

in the fog
for a friend coming out of the fog
I keep waiting

- Seisensui Ogiwara -

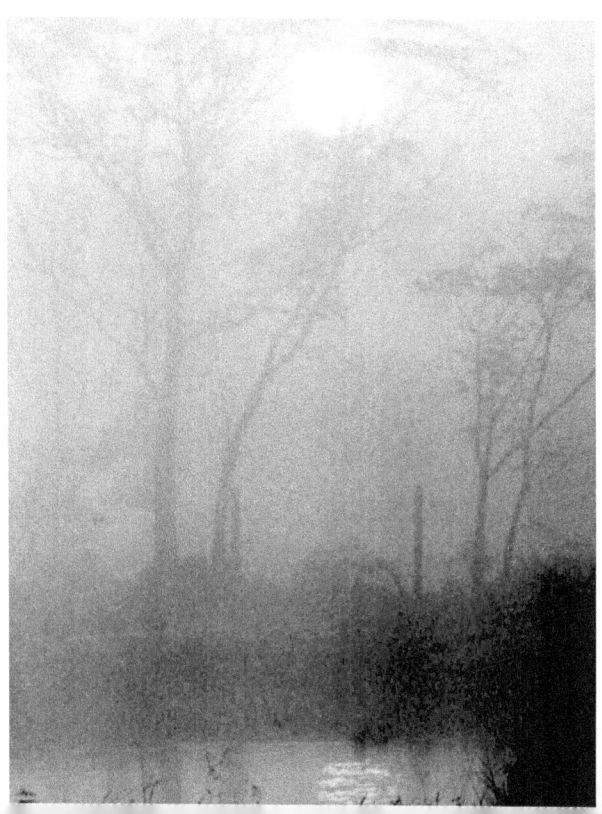

In this chapter, you will learn:

- How our understanding of meridians is changing.

- How the TCM meridian chart represents a simplified view of energy pathways.

- How each Regular Meridian actually has three routes.

Chapter 1

The Regular Meridians Revisited

The Traditional Chinese Medicine (TCM) chart of meridians and acupuncture points has become a symbol of Oriental medicine. It is an invaluable tool for practitioners visualizing and working with the patterns of energy flow throughout the human body. However, it is rarely acknowledged that this energy road map is a simplified version of a far more complex web of routes. Some information has been left out deliberately for practical reasons as we will discuss; some information has been forgotten over time or abandoned in the wake of cultural and political evolution and revolution; and much information awaits discovery.

While the TCM chart outlines essential points along the 12 Regular or main meridians and includes the Conception and Governing vessels, it ultimately leaves out far more than it includes. It does not address, for example, a multitude of anomalies in the points as they appear along the meridians, or irregularities in the meridians themselves as they transit the body from head to foot.

The TCM chart reveals nothing at all of the relationships between the Regular Meridians and other major meridian systems not on the chart — the Extra, Divergent, Ocean, and Cosmic systems. And while the detail presented on the standard TCM chart may be adequate for many acupuncturists, shiatsu therapists and other practitioners who focus upon the body's subtle energy systems would benefit greatly from a more precise knowledge of this much vaster meridian network. This could take Oriental medicine's focus well beyond the current emphasis on treatment with needles, and in doing so, greatly enhance the potential of our work.

The TCM Acupuncture Chart: An Efficient Shorthand

The TCM acupuncture chart we are familiar with today is based upon Katsupaku Jin's revisionary *Juyon Kei Raku Hatsuki* (*an Elucidation of Fourteen Meridians*), published in 1341. He is better known to the Chinese as Hua Shou, and his treatise, as *Shi-si Jing Hui*. Still an essential guide for understanding the energy flow of the human body, the chart illustrates specific acupuncture points along fixed pathways. It presents us with what appears to be a series of distinct, threadlike lines running vertically throughout the body: these represent the Regular Meridians — six channels on the arms and six on the legs — as well as two Extra Meridians on the torso. Especially in the energetically complex areas of the head and around the ankles, the illustrated pathways depart abruptly from their linear tendency to zigzag or circle in tight loops. I had often wondered how these awkward lines could be a true rendering of "natural" energy pathways.

It turns out I have not been alone in questioning the veracity or usefulness of these skinny, erratic lines. A growing chorus in the field of meridian research argues that energy actually travels via a relatively wide band comprised of three parallel channels flowing throughout the body.

What I have come to appreciate in the course of my own research is that this is one of many adaptations that appear on the charts we see today, and that such adaptations exist for the laudable purpose of simplicity. Wide, complex, and layered routes have been converted into an efficient shorthand for busy practitioners using needles. That this shorthand is so extensive, consistent, and thorough is testimony to just how comprehensive the original bank of Chinese medical knowledge must have been, and how farsighted the meridian chart's originators were.

It is hard to imagine a single chart illustrating the body's multiple meridian systems, their interrelationships, point conjunctions, and connections. That the sages of long ago untangled the web and designed a map of the essentials is an accomplishment that remains unsurpassed to this day.

Creating, or re-creating, a more complete picture of the human energy matrix is much like going on an archeological dig. We have pieces of information in hand; we know key pieces are missing. What was known? What waits to be discovered? Putting it all together falls to us.

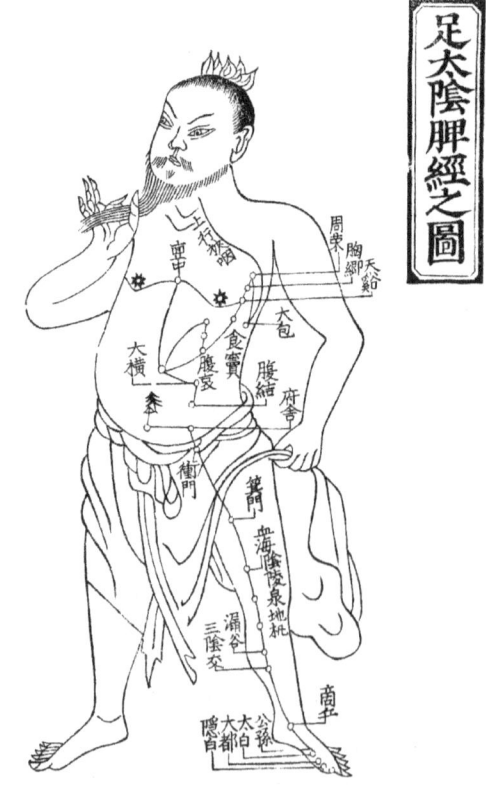

Figure 1-1 Spleen Meridian illustrated by Katsupaku Jin (Hua Shou), as published in 1341

The Twelve Meridians:
Three Levels of Imbalance

The classics acknowledge what the TCM chart does not and cannot show. Each of the 12 Regular Meridians can manifest at a first, second, or third level of imbalance, with the latter reflecting the deepest or most chronic level of illness. Further, at each of these levels, the meridian will shift its position: in other words, it will flow along a slightly different pathway.

First-level Imbalance: 平脈
Hei-myaku (Normal State)

As long as we are alive, no matter how healthy we feel, we will always experience some degree of energetic disharmony. Our body's various systems are always exerting themselves to maintain homeostasis, and this effort is reflected in the meridian system. So, even when our body is relatively "well balanced," we can still detect signs of compensation in the meridians. In shiatsu, energetic disharmony is described in terms of kyo and jitsu, where kyo represents a deficient, quieted, or slowed quality of energy, and jitsu reflects a relatively excessive or quickened quality.

The hei-myaku state represents the first level of imbalance, yet it is also what we would describe as the most normal energy state. This means that a subtle disharmony exists even though there may be no symptoms or signs of disease. We would, ideally, find a "natural imbalance" in which both the Stomach and Kidney meridians are kyo, and the Liver and Large Intestine meridians are jitsu. This particular pattern seems to reflect the deeply significant role of these four meridians in absorbing, creating, and refining ki in the body (see Chapter 4). While in the hei-myaku state, these meridians (and the remaining eight Regular Meridians) will maintain their normal, first-degree flow patterns.

Second-level Imbalance: 是動病
Ze-do-byo (Meridian Disease)

When greater demands are made on the meridian system — for example, if it tries to fight off a pathogen, accommodate mental or emotional stress, or correct some bodily weakness — then its level of imbalance deepens. In this case, the meridians mainly charged with correcting this imbalance will start to flow in their second-degree pathways. The imbalance has "spilled over" into the second degree,

TCM		Shin So Shiatsu
Hei-myaku 平脈 Normal, balanced	a	First-degree imbalance
Ze-do-byo 是動病 Meridian disease	b	Second-degree imbalance
Sho-sei-byo 所生病 Organ disease	c	Third-degree imbalance

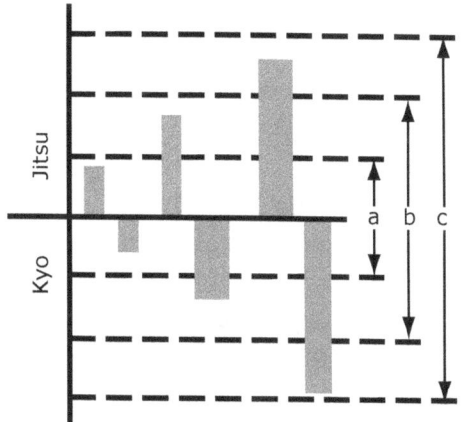

Figure 1-2 The three levels of Regular Meridian imbalance as denoted in the TCM and Shin So Shiatsu systems respectively

a condition known as ze-do-byo, or "meridian disease." The imbalance may not necessarily be deep enough to affect our zang-fu organs, yet we will certainly feel some symptoms.

We can liken the different pathways of a single meridian to wires with different capacities for handling electricity. When an imbalance is more than the first-degree pathways can handle, it spills over into second degree, engaging the higher-capacity pathways of the second-degree flow. This is not an exact metaphor: we cannot say at this time that meridians in second degree handle a "greater current" or "higher vibration" than first-degree channels. However, it is clear that the activation of second-degree pathways represents an increased level of activity on the part of the meridian system — a stronger effort to restore harmonious functioning to the organism.

When the meridian system is in the ze-do-byo state, we will find one second-degree meridian to be kyo, and one to be jitsu. The other 10 meridians however, will maintain their first-degree flow pattern.

Third-level Imbalance: 所生病 Sho-sei-byo (Organ Disease)

This is the deepest level of disharmony within the Regular Meridian system. When an imbalance requires more energy to be brought to bear on it than the second-degree channels can accommodate, the imbalance will "spill over" into the third-degree pathways. Again this will manifest in one third-degree meridian exhibiting a kyo state, and another a jitsu state: this imbalance is more clearly apparent than in the first two levels.

Patients with a sho-sei-byo imbalance still may not present a clinically detectable organ illness: this depends upon the nature of the imbalance and the individual. Yet this is seen as a deeper level of disharmony, one closer to directly involving the internal organs, and thus described as "organ disease."

What the Classics Say

The classics of Oriental medicine distinguish symptoms that might be experienced at these three levels. For example, a patient with the Kidney Meridian at the ze-do-byo (meridian-disease) level, may experience poor appetite, darker face color, bad cough with blood, eye problems, an unclear mind, and fear. At the sho-sei-byo (organ-disease) level, symptoms might progress to include heat sensations in the mouth, swelling, dryness, sore throat, diarrhea, hot sensations on the bottom of the feet, and cold sensations on the lower leg.

Although many of these tri-level symptoms have been documented, their integration into meridian-based treatments has been limited by our inability as therapists to appreciate exactly what the meridians are doing. What my research has been able to do is show is a clear correlation between this body of theoretical knowledge and the behavior of meridians in the body.

Toward a More Complete Picture

The TCM chart presents *portions* of the meridians, largely as they appear in their first-degree, or normal state. A few segments of the chart reflect what I have identified as second- or third-degree flows, but these are not specified as such. In other words, the TCM chart is a convenient shorthand for a much more complex energy matrix. Moving toward a more comprehensive view of the body's energy flow, we must look to more contemporary research.

Shizuto Masunaga:
A Great Leap Forward

Shizuto Masunaga's controversial Shiatsu Meridian Chart, published in the 1960s, was a major departure from the TCM chart which was until then gospel to Japanese and Chinese therapists working with energy. I had the good fortune to study with Masunaga at the Japan Shiatsu College in Tokyo between 1966 and 1968.

Masunaga was born in Hiroshima Prefecture in 1925, to a family of shiatsu practitioners. He studied psychology at Kyoto University, then stepped into the field of shiatsu to become one of the most gifted therapists of his day. For 10 years he taught psychology at the Japan Shiatsu College under Tokujiro Namikoshi, while continuing his own studies under Dr. Fusajiro Kato, a highly respected psychiatric doctor and pioneer in the field of occupational therapy. He then founded the Iokai Center to teach his own evolving shiatsu approach.

Masunaga's studies in psychology had a deep impact on his approach to shiatsu. He recognized both the physical and psychological components of energy imbalances, and explored these connections in his published work. He brought many other innovations to shiatsu, including supplementation and sedation via the use of two hands, the categorizing of meridian imbalances in terms of kyo and jitsu (broadly: "deficient" and "excess"), and a protocol of meridian imagery exercises. Yet it is his expanded network of meridians, illustrated in his chart, which has been his most significant and controversial legacy.

Masunaga possessed three qualities that made him a genius in the field of meridian research and treatment. He had

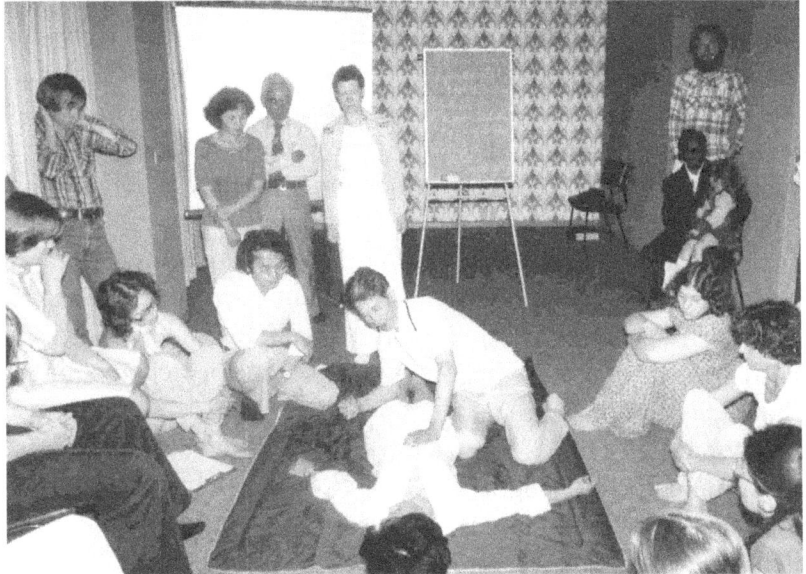

Figure 1-3 Shizuto Masunaga in Toronto, Canada in 1980. Ted Saito is immediately to his right.

an insatiable appetite for the classics of Oriental medicine and, right up to the end of his life, cherished every minute he could spend with them. Masunaga's mastery of this literature nourished his passion for clinical research. In this, he set himself apart from his peers who were mainly concerned with transferring the existing system of acupuncture points and meridians into shiatsu practice.

He wrote: "For a long time I was trying to find a pattern in the systemic responses of my patients. Just when I thought I had it, I was astounded to find that it already existed in ancient China in the form of meridians. However, the more I researched meridians, the more I came to realize that the classical meridian approach was a convenient shorthand for acupuncture treatment."

It was Masunaga's third and perhaps most unusual capacity that empowered his relentless hands-on exploration of ki and meridians, and shiatsu's influence upon them. Masunaga possessed what we call *meijin-gei* in Japanese, "master's skill," the rare ability to sense ki as it flows through the meridians. He could feel the complex relationships between meridians, and was able to diagnose the condition of the whole body from the hara. I once asked Masunaga's wife, Keiko Masunaga, how he did this — whether she recalled him developing his sensitivity through any particular techniques such as meditation or qi gong. She recalled none.

Masunaga's work crystallized into his own Zen Shiatsu system. His chart — with its 12 meridians running the full length of the body and unique hara (abdominal) diagnostic system — was an instant sensation. I remember many heated debates over whether or not Masunaga's "new" routes existed. Yet, despite initial skepticism, Masunaga's chart has remained central to a popular and enduring meridian-based shiatsu approach.

Between 1975 and 1980, Masunaga made regular visits to Canada to teach workshops at The Shiatsu Centre I had just established in Toronto. Shiatsu was as new and exotic as acupuncture to North Americans, and a handful of energetic young practitioners, also new to the West, were engaged in the monumental task of building its reputation. We had little to offer Masunaga in payment for his visits or even his travel expenses, but he continued to journey halfway around the globe to support his students and share what he knew.

What I heard most from Masunaga during those times was the importance of developing a high level of diagnostic skill. He felt this was what distinguished a professional from an unprofessional therapist. Without a strong foundation in Oriental medical theory and a good working knowledge of the meridian system, he explained, a therapist could not properly diagnose or provide effective treatment. "It is not important how many hours one has studied," he once told me, "or even how many years one has practiced. It is the manner of study enabling strong diagnostic ability that matters." Beyond this, he believed students must be trained to sense, communicate with, and diagnose through the meridians.

My deep appreciation for Masunaga Sensei and the depth of his insights fuels my commitment to continue with the work he began but was unable to finish before his untimely death in 1981.

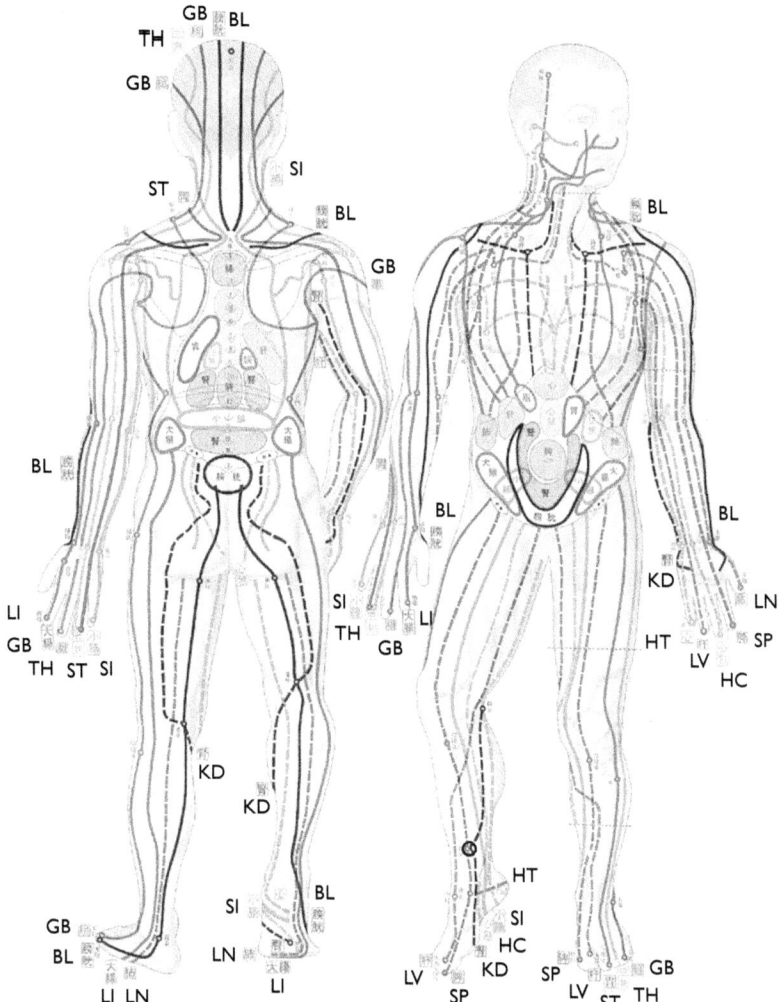

Figure 1-4a Masunaga's meridian chart was published in the 1960s: only now are some of its mysteries being resolved.

Meridian Name	Abbreviation	Meridian Name	Abbreviation
Lung	LN	Large Intestine	LI
Spleen	SP	Stomach	ST
Heart	HT	Small Intestine	SI
Kidney	KD	Bladder	BL
Heart Constrictor	HC	Triple Heater	TH
Liver	LV	Gallbladder	GB
Governor	GV	Conception	CV

Figure 1-4b Abbreviation of meridian names

Beyond Zen Shiatsu:
Saito Regular Meridians

While Masunaga's controversial system represented what I believed to be a much more complete picture of the human energy matrix than the TCM chart, it remained unproven and unexplained in the years following his death. With Dr. Tadashi Irie's Finger Test Method (see Chapter 3) and its potential for locating energy pathways, I took on the task of exploring and charting the Regular Meridians for myself. It became readily apparent that not just one, but three distinctive pathways existed for each of the 12 Regular Meridians. This supported what I had read in the classics, and led me to the astonishing discovery, mentioned above, that meridian pathways will shift in a very particular pattern depending on the level of imbalance within the energy system.

I was able to draw detailed charts for each of the three levels. When I compared my findings with Masunaga's, I realized that for the most part he had drawn the Regular Meridians as they would appear at the third, or deepest, level of disharmony. In a few small instances, his rendition overlaps with what I would consider to be the second level of disharmony.

Figure 1-5a shows us how closely Masunaga's pathway for the Large Intestine Meridian compares to that meridian in third-degree as I have charted it (figure 1-5d and 1-5e). Figures 1-5b and 1-5c illustrate first- and second-degree flows for the Large Intestine Meridian.

Why had Masunaga charted only the third level? I recalled him saying that, despite his sensitivity, it had not been easy to map the energy flow for the entire body. Knowingly or unknowingly, perhaps, he chose models with more serious health problems, whose more imbalanced meridian flows were easier for him to sense. Perhaps also, he knew that if the more serious third level was addressed, the other two levels would regulate automatically, and thus his priority would have been to present the third level in chart form to his students.

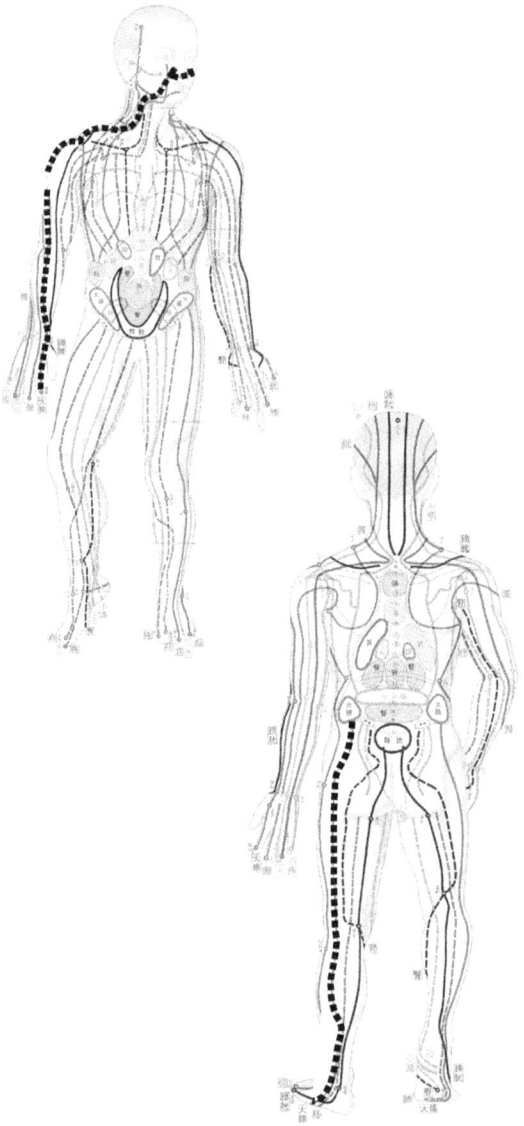

Figure 1-5a Masunaga's pathway for the Large Intestine Meridian is shown as a dotted line.

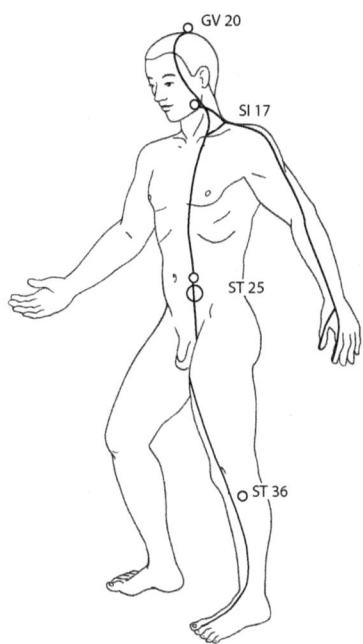

Figure 1-5b Saito Large Intestine Meridian: first-degree flow

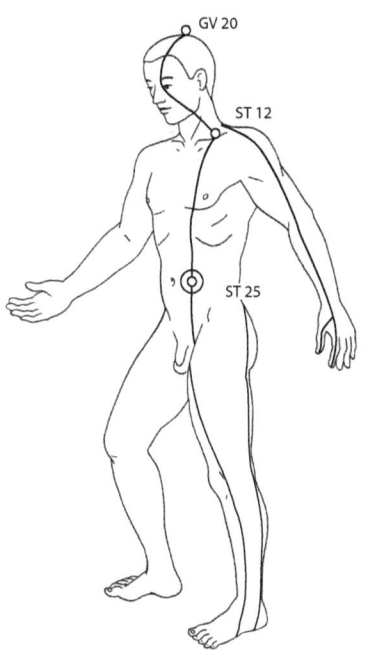

Figure 1-5d Saito Large Intestine Meridian: third-degree flow

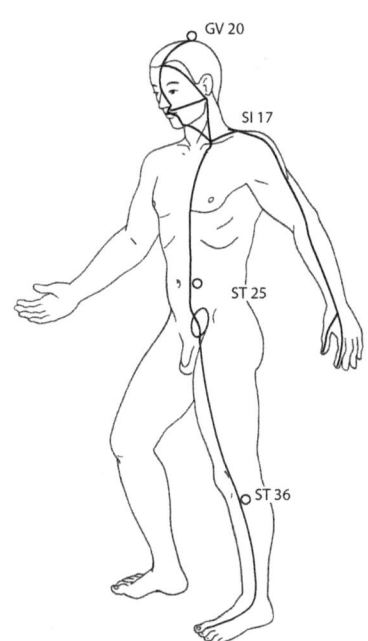

Figure 1-5c Saito Large Intestine Meridian: second-degree flow

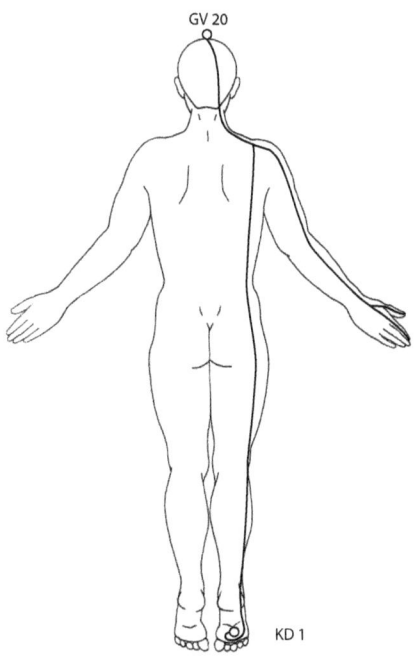

Figure 1-5e Saito Large Intestine Meridian: third-degree flow

Regular Meridians Up Close

As earlier mentioned, TCM meridians appear as single, narrow lines of energy running throughout the body. My research has confirmed not only that three pathways exist for each meridian (corresponding to the three levels of imbalance), but also that each of these three pathways exists as three parallel lines — where each line represents an area of higher energy density and the spaces between these lines represent areas of much lower density. This concurs with findings published by Dr. Rokuro Fujita and Tsutomu Kishi, Dr. Ac. (*An Introduction to Meridianology*, So Gen-Sha, Osaka, Japan, 1980).

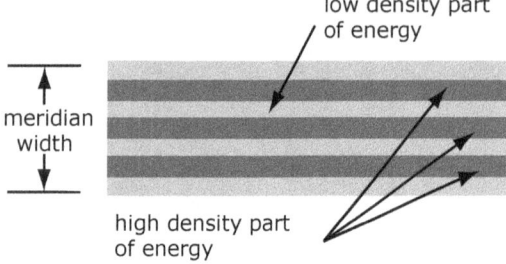

Figure 1-6a A meridian

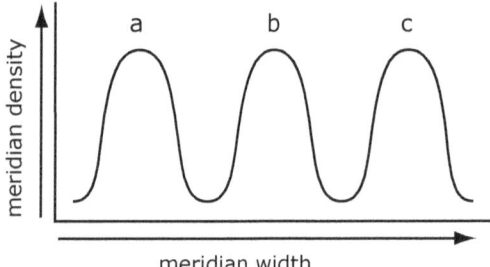

Figure 1-6b Profile of a meridian

Figure 1-6a and 1-6b illustrate these varying energy densities relative to the total meridian width. Points a, b, and c represent the higher density areas, easily detected with the Finger Test Method.

Figure 1-7 illustrates the three lines of the Stomach Meridian on the lateral aspect of the leg.

My research also supports Fujita and Kishi in their observation that acupuncture points are situated along all three of these parallel lines, as shown in figure 1-8.

The energy density, or diameter, of acupuncture points also varies: some points overlap onto other lines, as shown in figure 1-9.

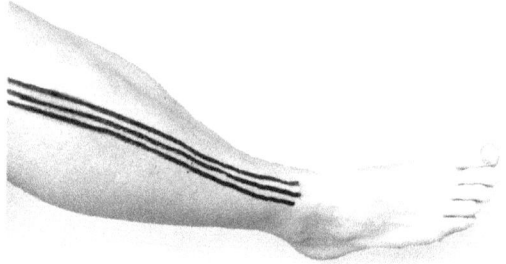

Figure 1-7 Stomach Meridian

Figure 1-10 illustrates how acupuncture points might appear along the three parallel lines of any given meridian.

We can see how cleaning up what seem to be superfluous lines on the meridian pathway results in the TCM chart's distinctive point-to-point sketch of the body's energy flow. To create this leaner and easy-to-read chart, two lines have been

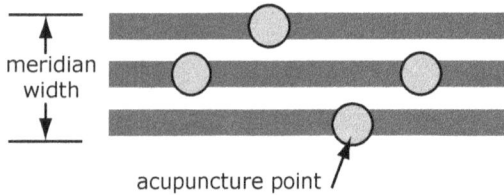

Figure 1-8

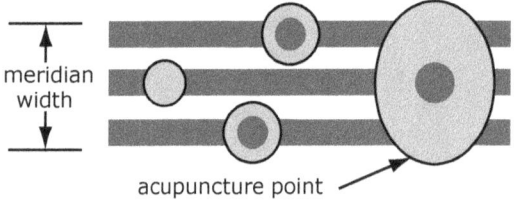

Figure 1-9

eliminated. But, since many important and effective acupuncture points are situated on the eliminated lines, a single-lined illustration would result in the unnatural looking flow illustrated in figure 1-11.

Drawing a line that connects these acupuncture points creates the zigzags and loops characteristic of the TCM chart. This is most apparent for the Gallbladder, Small Intestine, Stomach, and Triple Heater meridians, as illustrated in figure 1-12.

Figure 1-13 shows the Kidney Meridian as it appears on the TCM chart and as it appears with three parallel lines of energy flow. The TCM chart's Kidney Meridian loops below the ankle, but in our bodies, it flows more naturally, as a stream would.

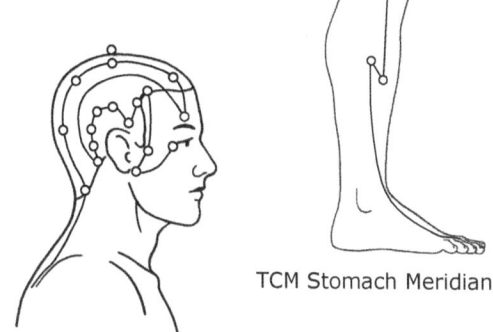

TCM Gallbladder Meridian

TCM Stomach Meridian

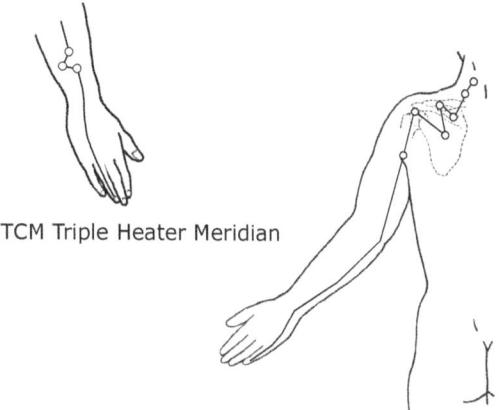

TCM Triple Heater Meridian

TCM Small Intestine Meridian

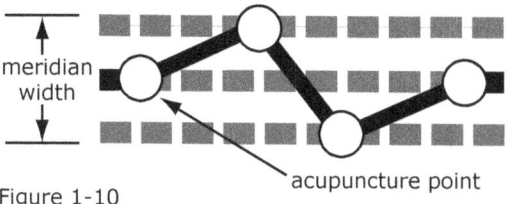

Figure 1-10

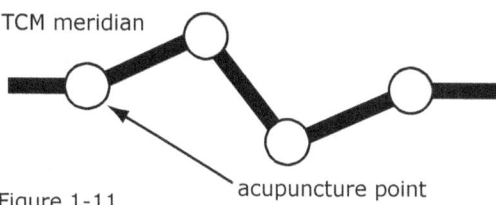

Figure 1-11

Figure 1-12 These four TCM meridians follow particularly erratic routes.

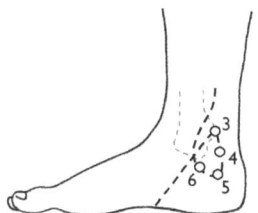

Figure 1-13a TCM Kidney Meridian

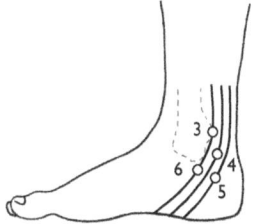

Figure 1-13b Saito Kidney Meridian

Figure 1-14a
Gallbladder Meridian as it appears on the TCM chart

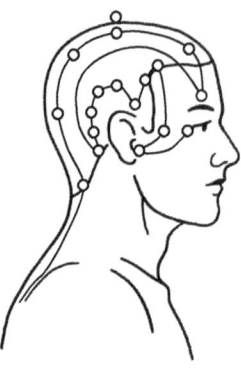

Figure 1-14b
Gallbladder Meridian as it appears on the Saito Meridian Charts in each of the first, second, and third degrees

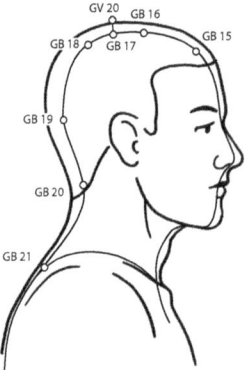

First-degree flow

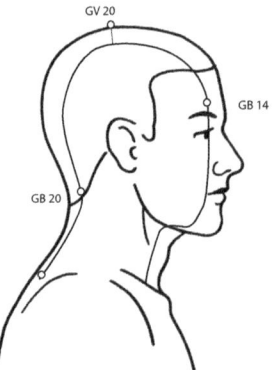

Second-degree flow

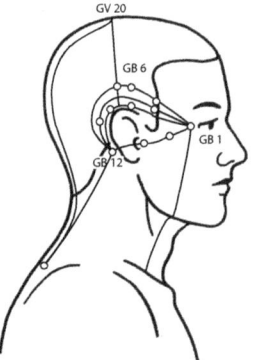

Third-degree flow

An Overview of TCM Simplifications

While each of the 12 meridians run the body's full length, the TCM chart presents only portions of the external pathways, so it appears that only six meridians flow on the upper body and six on the lower body.

- Only the exterior portions of the meridians, and not their internal branches, are illustrated on the TCM chart.

- While the energy of each meridian flows in three parallel lines, the TCM chart illustrates only one line, but incorporates onto that key points from the other two lines.

- While there are three levels of energy flow — and hence distinct lines of flow for each level — the TCM chart shows us mostly the first level and primarily points associated with the first level. In a few instances, however, acupuncture points for all three levels of imbalance have been incorporated onto one line, adding to the appearance of a zigzagged pathway. A good example of this is the distribution of the Gallbladder Meridian on the side of the head, as in figure 1-14.

While the ancients likely understood that a complexity of points lay along a multi-dimensional course, the TCM chart leaves us with a very two-dimensional view. Here are a few more examples:

- We know yin energy normally ascends, but information missing on the TCM chart leads to the impression that Spleen energy descends from SP 20 to SP 21.

- The TCM chart does not show how the Spleen Meridian connects to the Spleen Bo Point (Front Mu Point) at LV 13. My research shows that in the case of a third-degree imbalance, the Spleen Meridian connects to LV 13.

- The Small Intestine and Stomach meridians are far more complex than the TCM chart suggests, as seen in figures 1-15 and 1-16.

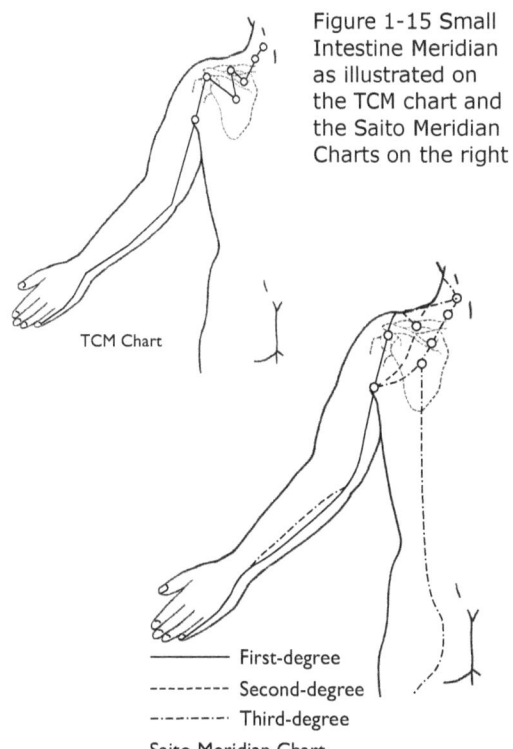

Figure 1-15 Small Intestine Meridian as illustrated on the TCM chart and the Saito Meridian Charts on the right

Where They Flow:
The Regular Meridians in General

We can make the following generalizations about the flow patterns for the Regular Meridians in the human body:

- All 12 Regular Meridians flow throughout the whole body.

- Regardless of the degree of imbalance, all six yang Regular meridians begin at GV 20 and at the fingertips, and end at KD 1. All six yin Regular meridians begin at KD 1 and end at GV 20 as well as the fingertips.

- All 12 Regular Meridians flow through the eyes.

- All six yin meridians pass through the genital region.

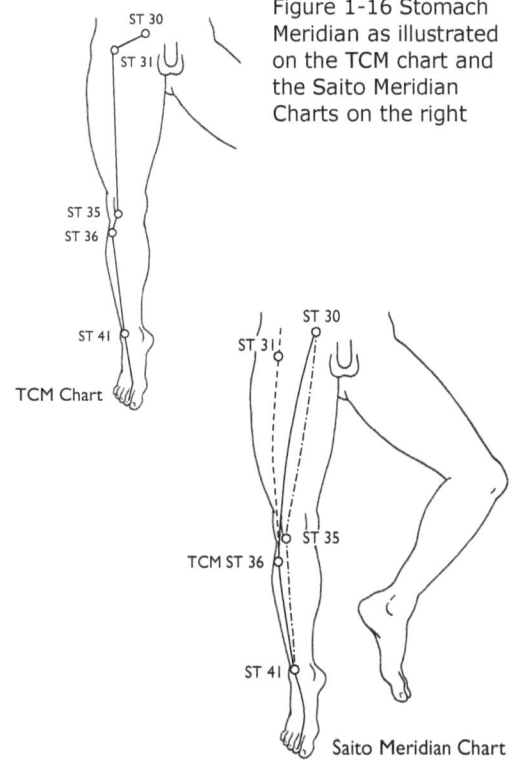

Figure 1-16 Stomach Meridian as illustrated on the TCM chart and the Saito Meridian Charts on the right

Yin Regular Meridians in First and Second Degree

From KD 1, the yin meridians run up and inside the leg. From the inner thigh, below the genitals, the energy branches into two divisions. One branch overlaps the Conception Vessel and flows along this meridian to

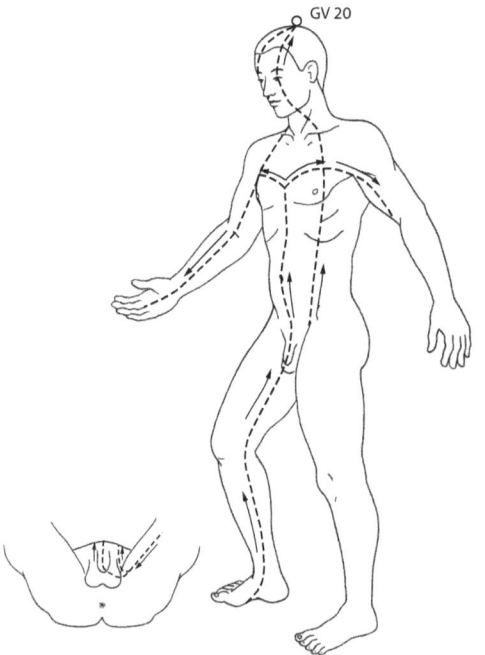

Figure 1-17 General flow of yin Regular Meridians in first and second degree (Saito Meridian Charts)

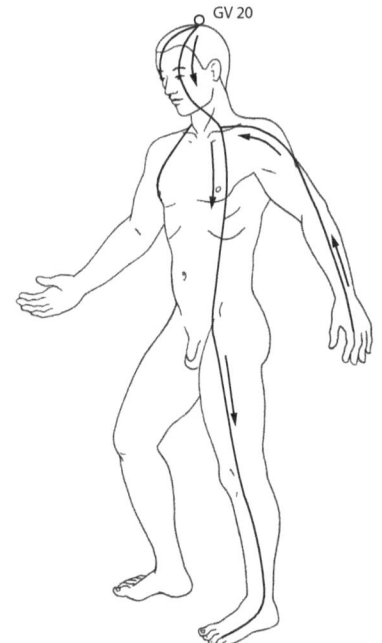

Figure 1-18 General flow of yang Regular Meridians in first and second degree (Saito Meridian Charts)

the chest, then branches to the arms and runs to the fingertips where the meridians end. The second branch flows from the abdomen, to the chest, neck, and face, finishing at the top of the head at GV 20.

The pathway of this first branch differs slightly in men and women. In males, the first branch flows into the scrotum, then into the root of the penis, looping down the posterior and then up the anterior side of the penis before following the Conception Vessel up the abdomen. In women, this flow will go to the clitoris and then travels via the Conception Vessel to the navel, and up via the Penetrating Meridian.

Yang Regular Meridians in First and Second Degree

Energy from the yin meridians transfers to the yang meridians at GV 20 and the fingertips where the yin meridians end. The yang energy from the fingertips runs along the posterior aspect of the arm to the shoulder, where it meets with the yang energy that has descended through the face, neck, and shoulder from GV 20. These two branches join, and descend as one energy flow through the chest, abdomen, leg and foot, ending at KD 1. The one exception is the Bladder Meridian, which manifests a flow along the dorsal side of the body, but only in its second-degree flow, not in first degree. No yang meridian transits the back of the body in first degree.

Yin Regular Meridians in Third Degree

The pathways for the yin meridians in first or second degree are very similar, appearing only on the body's ventral aspect, not the dorsal. When the imbalance advances to the third degree, however, the energy flow appears at both ventral and dorsal aspects of the body.

Again, all yin meridians begin at KD 1 and flow up the inner thigh, but from here the flow branches into three directions as follows:

- One branch begins near the genital region and follows a pattern similar to the yin Regular Meridians in first- and second-degree states. That is to say, one branch runs with the Conception Vessel (in men; with the Conception Vessel and then Penetrating Vessel in women) before splitting to run into the arms, while another runs up the torso to end at GV 20.

- One branch flows up the leg medially and into GV 1, then flows diagonally up the back and around the chest to reconnect with the branch running up the ventral part of the torso.

- A third branch runs parallel to the spine from GV 1 to GV 20.

In observing the third-degree flow for yin meridians, several interesting details emerge, some of which help us to make more sense of the TCM chart, while others help us to understand issues which puzzled those who studied Masunaga's early chart. For example:

- In the course of my research, questions have arisen regarding Bo points or Mu points. For example, as I trace the Large Intestine Meridian in third degree, I can sense the Large Intestine Meridian Bo Point in its classical location at ST 25.

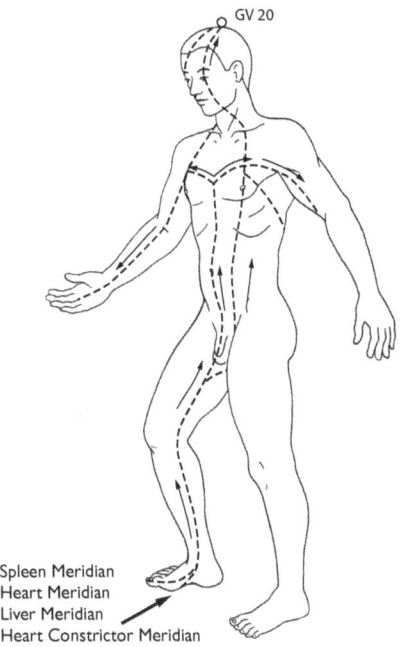

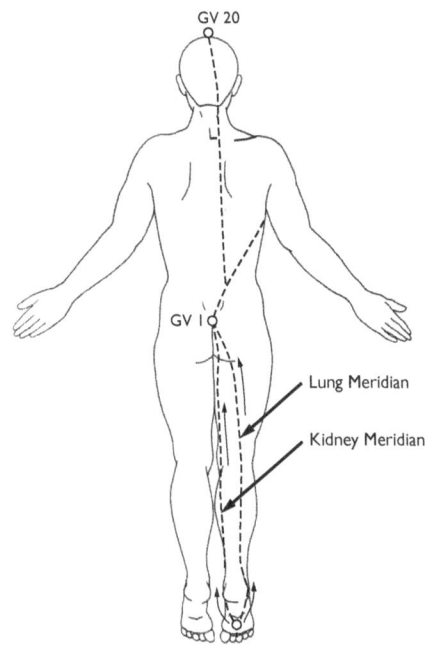

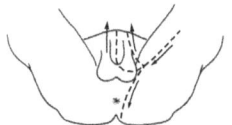

Figure 1-19 General flow of yin Regular Meridians in third-degree (Saito Meridian Charts)

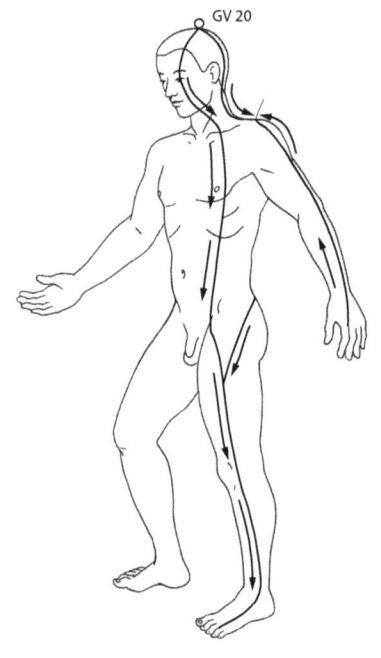

Strangely however, while TCM theory puts the Kidney Bo Point on the Gallbladder Meridian at GB 25, I have been unable to sense any Kidney Meridian energy there. I have found that when the Kidney Meridian reaches the third degree of imbalance, KD 16 begins to vibrate, activating the third-degree hara diagnostic zone.

- It is also important to note that both the Kidney and Lung meridians in the third degree flow along the posterior, not the medial side of the upper leg. Looking at Masunaga's chart, we see how similar his trajectories are for these meridians. Figure 1-19 illustrates the general flow of the yin Regular Meridians in third degree.

Yang Regular Meridians in Third Degree

- All of the yang meridians begin at GV 20 as well as the fingertips, where the yin meridians end. From the top of the head at GV 20, the energy branches in two directions.

- The first branch, beginning at GV 20, follows the anterior aspect of the face, through the eye, neck, chest, and abdomen, travelling to the leg and foot, ending at KD 1. The portion of the meridian beginning at the fingertips follows the posterior aspect of the arm to the shoulder.

- A second branch, from GV 20, descends the posterior of the head to the neck and shoulder. At the shoulder, it connects with the yang energies rising from the fingertips, and as one flow, travels

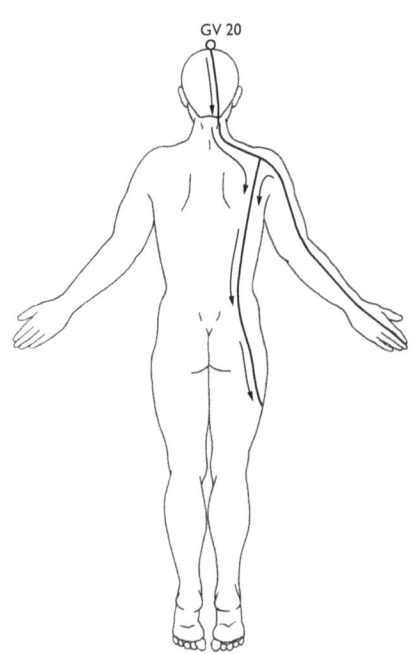

Figure 1-20 General flow of yang Regular Meridians in third-degree (Saito Meridian Charts)

down the back, to the hip and leg. This flow travels around the buttocks and upper thigh to connect with the former branch, beginning at GV 20, that runs down the anterior aspect of the body. These two flows reconnect at a particular point (depending on the meridian) along the antero-lateral aspect of the thigh and lower leg, and travel together along the lower leg to end at KD 1. See figure 1-20.

Once we understand how third-degree energy flow manifests in distinct pathways on the back, it becomes clearer why this part of the body tends to "speak out more" in cases of serious or chronic illness. It is only when an imbalance reaches the third or "organ-disease" level, that the Regular Meridians manifest here. Hence, this becomes an essential area for rebalancing the meridians.

This phenomenon also sheds more light on the importance accorded the Bladder Meridian in acupuncture. Many significant points exits along this pathway, notably the back Transporting Points (Shu Points), which are considered to be directly related to organ function.

Yet this is clearly another simplification from the TCM chart. The Bladder Meridian is not the only Regular Meridian to transit the back of the body: all of the Regular Meridians do so when they reach a third-degree state of imbalance.

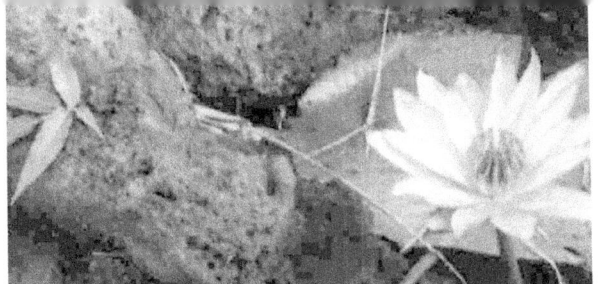

2

New Phenomena
Energy Circles and Meridian Belt Zones

seaside temple...
among the wood chips
irises

- Issa Kobayashi -

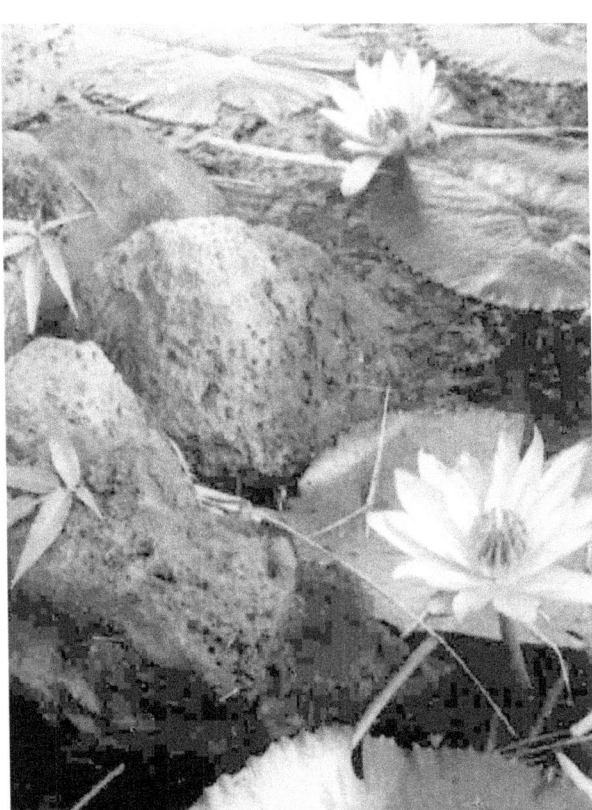

In this chapter, you will learn:

- How the meridian system is more than a series of linear pathways.

- How energy circles take many forms.

- How meridian belt zones help us locate meridian lines.

Chapter 2

New Phenomena
Energy Circles and Meridian Belt Zones

Using the Finger Test Method, I was able to develop a more extensive knowledge of the Regular Meridians than I had dreamed possible. But this was just the tip of the iceberg. As my meridian tracing skills increased, so did my sensitivity to other forms of energy.

I continued to explore lingering questions about Shizuto Masunaga's groundbreaking work, particularly his charts of the hara and back diagnostic zones. Although they had been in wide use since the early 1970s, they had not been fully explained or further developed. There were also his meridian stretch positions, faithfully adopted by a generation of therapists, although no one had satisfactorily clarified their relationship to the meridians.

As my research progressed, I found explanations for these puzzles in two unusual energetic phenomena. The first, energy circles — detectable circles of energy located anywhere on the surface of the body — provided me with a larger context for Masunaga's hara diagnostic zones. The second, meridian belt zones — bands of energy covering the entire body from head to toe — provided a context not only for Masunaga's back diagnostic zones, but also for his meridian stretch positions. Both play central roles in Shin So diagnosis and treatment.

Meridian Diagnostic Zones are Energy Circles

Anyone who has practiced Zen Shiatsu is familiar with Masunaga's chart of unusual hara diagnostic zones: a sea of elongated, sometimes overlapping "islands" covering the entire belly from sternum to pubis. It is here, in the abdomen, that the condition of the meridians is reflected. Hara diagnosis, so central to Zen Shiatsu, is somewhat similar to acupuncture's pulse assessment. Although, as I have mentioned, new students and well-seasoned therapists alike are challenged by the difficulties of mastering hara diagnosis by palpation.

My research, using the finger test to locate and map the Regular Meridians, led me quite naturally to a re-examination of Masunaga's meridian diagnostic zones on the hara. My own findings confirmed many aspects of Masunaga's chart, but I also uncovered some significant and helpful differences.

Three levels of Imbalance

Just as meridian locations shift with the degree of energy imbalance, so do hara diagnostic zones. Figure 2-1 shows us Masunaga's hara diagnostic chart; figures 2-2a, 2-2b, and 2-2c show the Saito hara diagnostic zones as they appear at all three levels of imbalance.

A closer look at the Masunaga and Saito abdominal charts turned up interesting correspondences. For instance, the Bladder and Kidney diagnostic zones on the Masunaga chart appear as U-shaped curves on the lower abdomen below the navel. On my charts, the same meridian zones appear more circular, and smaller. But when my tri-level charts are overlapped — so that we can see all three degrees of imbalance for the Bladder or Kidney zones in one image (see figures 2-3a and 2-3b) — Masunaga's overall pattern re-emerges (figure 2-3c). Whether or not he distinguished them, Masunaga was sensing all three levels as they curved under the navel area.

Masunaga's Large Intestine zone corresponds to my second-degree diagnostic zone for the Large Intestine. At this point, I cannot explain why he presented this particular view, nor can I explain our divergent views of the Small Intestine zone. Further research will no doubt shed more light on this.

I have found that most of the diagnostic zones for the yin organs that run along the lower costal area (LV, HT, HC, LN) shift upward from the hara to the mid- and upper chest as the level of imbalance increases. Conversely, the diagnostic zones for the yang organs shift down. Although there is no reference to these shifts on Masunaga's chart, I believe they reflect concepts of meridian- and organ-level disease understood by the ancients.

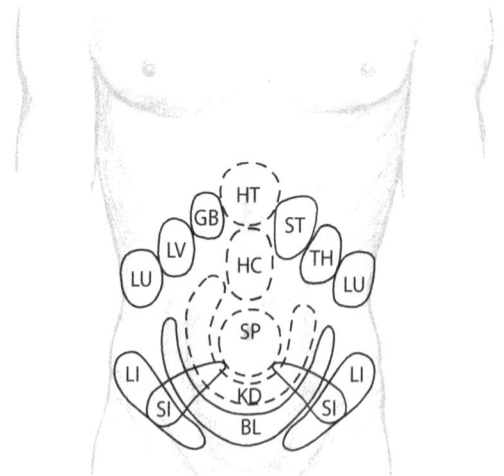

Figure 2-1 Masunaga's hara diagnostic chart

Shin So Shiatsu 35

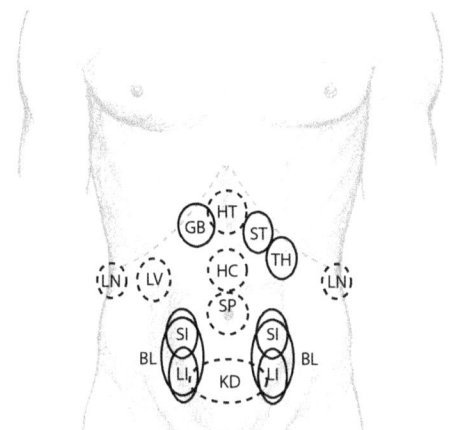

Figure 2-2a First-degree Regular Meridian imbalance (Saito diagnostic zones)

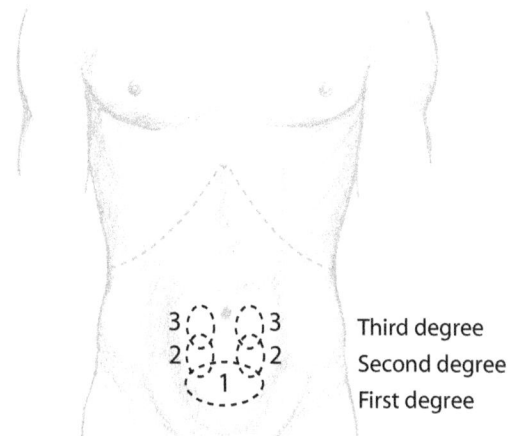

Figure 2-3a Saito Kidney Meridian zones

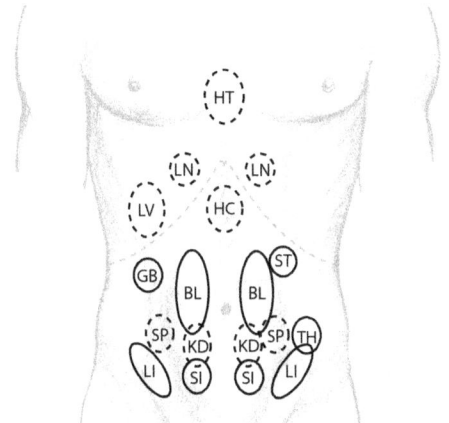

Figure 2-2b Second-degree Regular Meridian imbalance (Saito diagnostic zones)

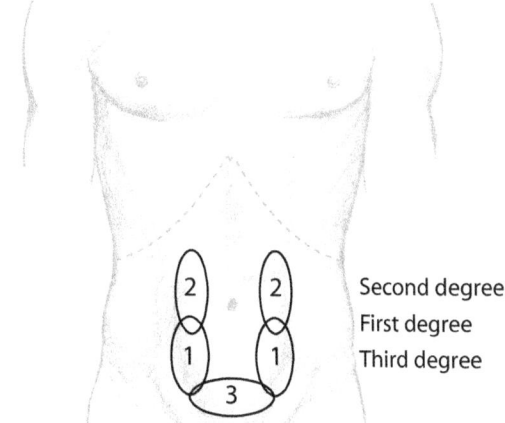

Figure 2-3b Saito Bladder Meridian zones

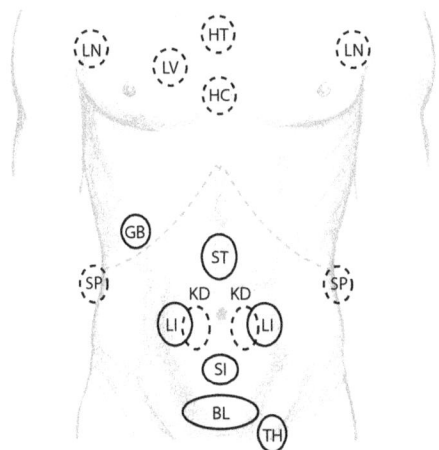

Figure 2-2c Third-degree Regular Meridian imbalance (Saito diagnostic zones)

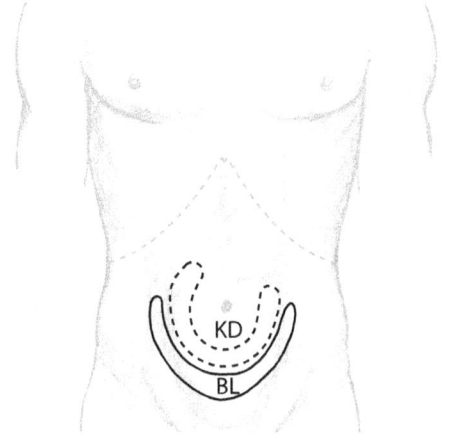

Figure 2-3c Masunaga's Bladder and Kidney diagnostic zones

Indeed, it is interesting to compare the Saito chart of the third-degree diagnostic zones with the TCM locations for Alarm (Bo or Front Mu) Points. While there is no obvious connection between these points and Masunaga's chart, a clear relationship begins to emerge when we see his zones shift to reflect deeper states of imbalance. Many of the third-degree zones on my chart coincide with the Front Mu Points. For example, when the Stomach Meridian is in a third-degree state, we can feel its energy in a circular zone around CV 12, the Alarm Point for the Stomach Meridian. This third-degree zone/Front Mu Point correspondence holds true for many meridians: Spleen, Lung, Large Intestine, Small Intestine, Bladder, Heart Constrictor, and Gallbladder.

There are some differences. For example, I find that the Liver Alarm Point corresponds to my second-degree Liver zone, and I locate the third-degree Kidney zone by the umbilicus, not on the side of the torso. Yet overall, the overlaps between my chart and the TCM distribution of Alarm Points strikes me as significant: it helps to harmonize shiatsu and TCM approaches, and again, is testimony to the great storehouse of knowledge developed by ancient Chinese.

Types of Energy Circles

I have come to appreciate that hara diagnostic zones fall under a larger category of energetic phenomena I call energy circles — detectable circles of energy that can be found anywhere on the surface of the body. Energy circles include:

1. The Regular Meridian diagnostic zones on the abdomen and chest for first-, second-, and third-degree imbalances.
2. Areas anywhere on the body's surface from head to foot reflecting structural problems that lie either superficially or at deeper, less palpable levels (chapters 4 and 6).
3. Circles reflecting imbalances in both the Extra and Divergent meridian systems (chapters 6 and 7).
4. Acupuncture points.

What these energy circles all have in common is that they represent areas where the body's energy system is asking — literally opening itself up — to receive help from the outside. Energy circles are areas of interchange between our energy system and the Cosmic energy system: where ja ki is "breathed out" and where sei ki is "breathed in" (for more about sei ki and ja ki, see Chapter 4).

Characteristics of Energy Circles

- The greater an energy imbalance, the larger the energy circle: the more severe or chronic an illness, i.e. the more help the body needs, the more area an energy circle will cover. (As you will see below, this phenomenon also holds true for meridian belt zones.) I believe this is associated with the meridian system's propensity to self regulate. The more disturbance a particular meridian experiences, the more sei ki it seeks to draw into its terrain, and the more accumulated ja ki it will discharge. Figures 2-4a and 2-4b illustrate how the Spleen Meridian diagnostic zone looks before and after treatment.

- Energy circles are holographic in nature: they reflect the condition of the whole body's energy system. Within the boundaries of an energy circle, we will be able to detect a number of vertical, horizontal, and diagonal lines. These will be vibrating with a specific quality of energy and direction of flow. The vertical lines appear to be associated with the Divergent Meridians, the deepest aspect of the Regular Meridian system, while the horizontal lines are associated with the Belt Meridian, which helps regulate all of the Extra Meridians. The diagonal lines are our link to the Cosmic energy system. Remarkably, as we shall see in later chapters, by treating such a small circular area of the body, we can support the whole body's energy system.

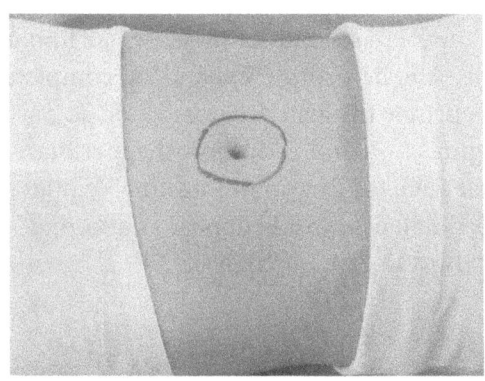

Figure 2-4a Spleen Meridian diagnostic zone before treatment

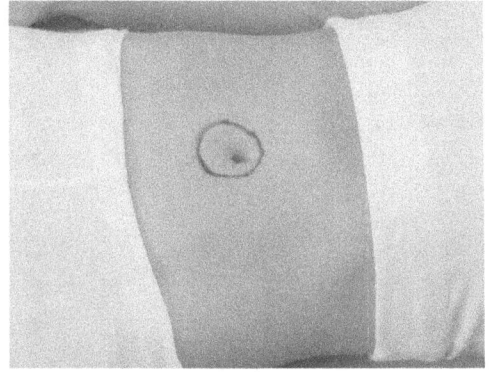

Figure 2-4b Spleen Meridian diagnostic zone after treatment

Meridian Belt Zones

In the early 1990s, my explorations with the finger test led to my exciting encounter with another new energetic phenomenon: belt-like energy zones covering the body's entire surface. I immediately realized that these "meridian belt zones," where they traverse the back torso, corresponded very closely to the reflex areas of Masunaga's back diagnostic chart. I also discovered that belt zones elsewhere on the body corresponded to the stretch positions Masunaga employed in his treatments. I will elaborate upon this central facet of Shin So Shiatsu below.

Realizing that such belt zones had never been reported before, I undertook to explore and map their boundaries in detail. They bore a certain resemblance to Kurakichi Hirata's well-known system of "Hirata zones." However, Hirata related his zones directly to the major anatomical organs of the body (see figure 2-5). My meridian belt zones clearly reflected meridian energetic functions. Later, in my work with the Divergent Meridian system, I would see the surprising confluence of Hirata's results and mine, described at the end of this chapter.

Characteristics of Meridian Belt Zones

Meridian belt zones are structurally unlike any other meridian. They are bands of energy encircling the arms, legs, torso and face. For each of these four regions of the body, there are 12 Regular Meridian belt zones, with each zone corresponding to a Regular Meridian. Meridian belt zones provide information about the degree of imbalance in the Regular Meridian system

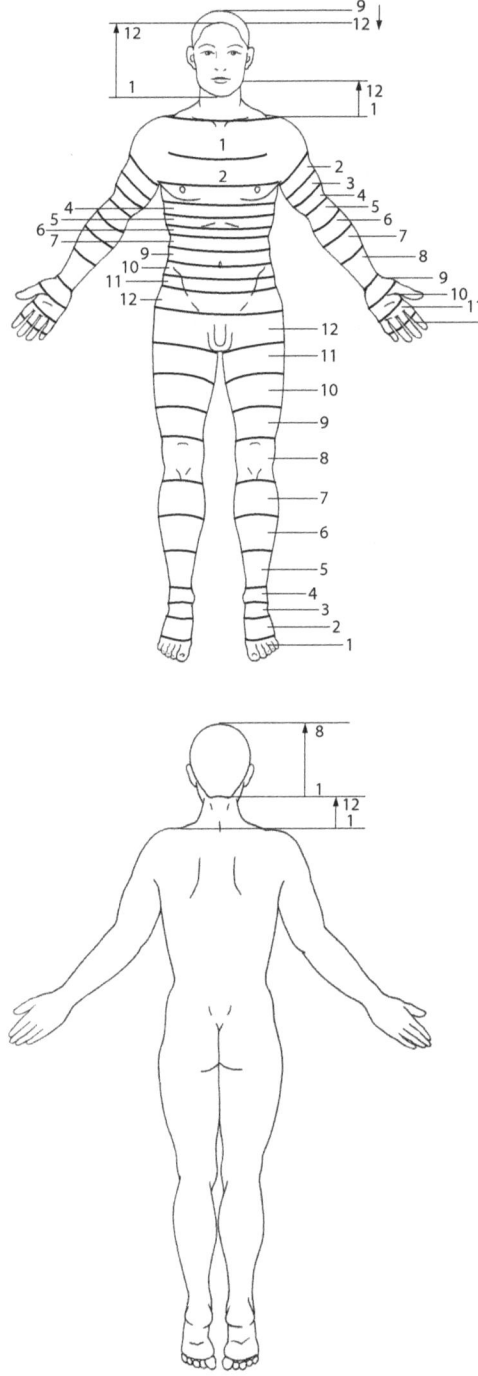

1 Trachea-bronchi
2 Lungs
3 Heart
4 Liver
5 Gallbladder
6 Spleen-pancreas
7 Stomach
8 Kidneys
9 Large Intestine
10 Small Intestine
11 Bladder
12 Genital organs

Figure 2-5 Hirata's Zones

and the kyo or jitsu nature of that imbalance. There are also belt zones corresponding to the Extra and Divergent meridian systems. Depending upon where they are situated on the body and which meridian system they reflect, their shape and size varies. Figures 2-6a and 2-6b illustrate the Regular Meridian belt zone on the arm for the Small Intestine in first degree.

We can see how the meridian belt zone at this normal energy level does not completely encircle the wrist. Using the finger test, we will sense the zone only on the radial portion of the wrist. This holds true for all Regular Meridian belt zones on all areas of the body reflecting a first-degree energy state: only a portion of the belt zone will appear active.

When the Regular Meridian system manifests a second- or third-degree imbalance, the belt zones "expand" to completely encircle the arm, leg, torso, and so on. Figures 2-7a and 2-7b show the meridian belt zone for the Small Intestine Regular Meridian as it would appear as a second- or third-degree imbalance.

Shin So Shiatsu 39

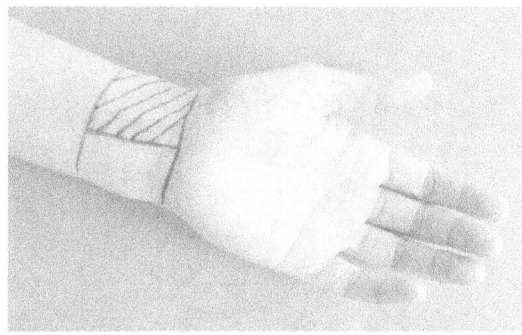

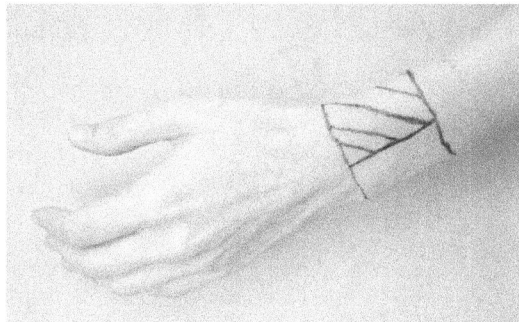

Figures 2-6a and 2-6b Small Intestine Meridian belt zone in normal energy state

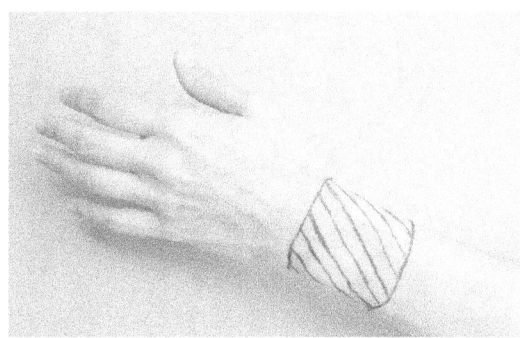

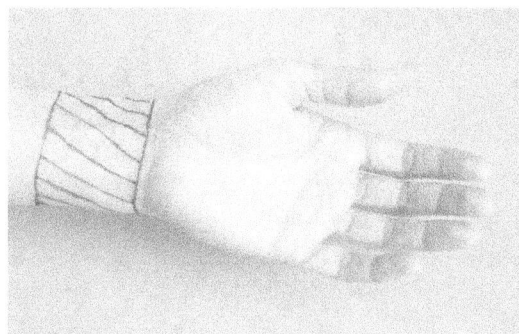

Figures 2-7a and 2-7b Small Intestine Regular Meridian belt zone in second- or third-degree imbalance

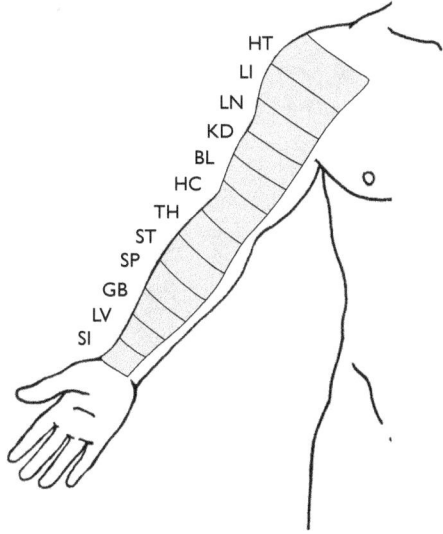

Figure 2-8a

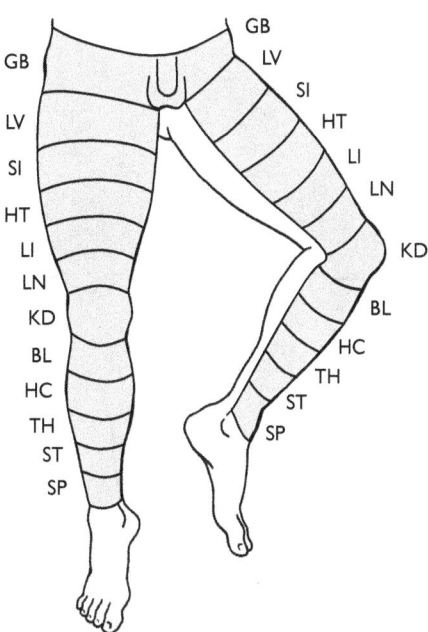

Figure 2-8b

Figures 2-8a to 2-8g The Regular Meridian belt zones in a first-degree or normal energy state. Belt zones on the arms and legs are similar in appearance to those of the belt zone shown in figures 2-7a and 2-7b, above, left. Belt zones on the chest and face are more rectangular in shape.

40 CHAPTER 2 NEW PHENOMENA: ENERGY CIRCLES AND MERIDIAN BELT ZONES

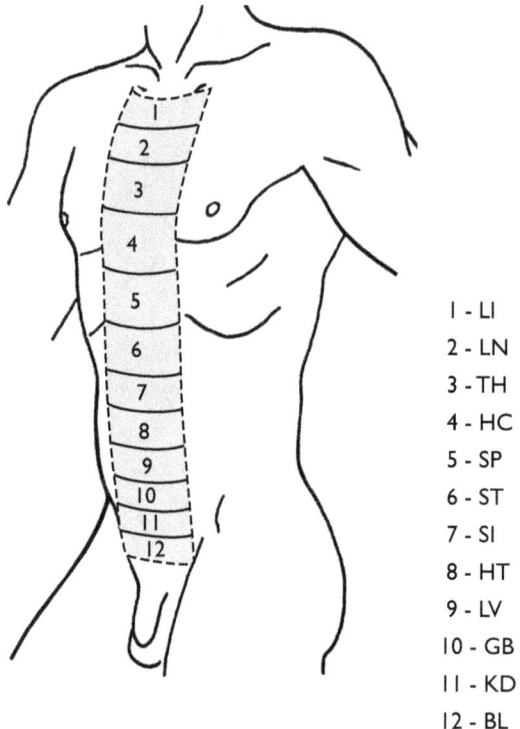

1 - LI
2 - LN
3 - TH
4 - HC
5 - SP
6 - ST
7 - SI
8 - HT
9 - LV
10 - GB
11 - KD
12 - BL

Figure 2-8c

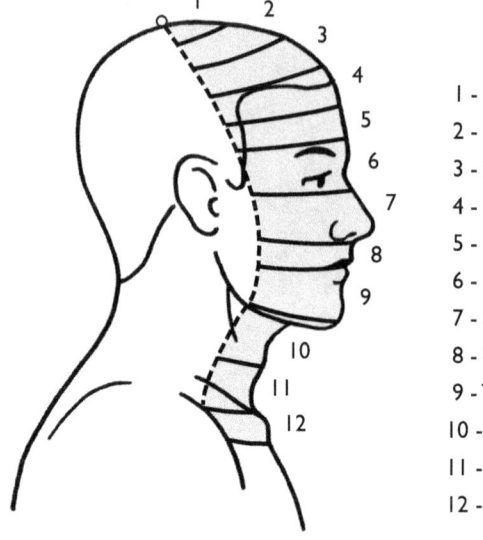

1 - BL
2 - KD
3 - SI
4 - HT
5 - GB
6 - LV
7 - SP
8 - ST
9 - TH
10 - HC
11 - LN
12 - LI

Figure 2-8e

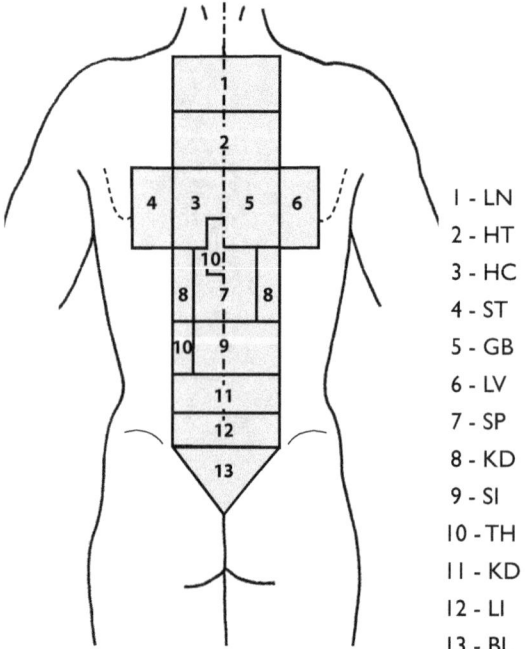

1 - LN
2 - HT
3 - HC
4 - ST
5 - GB
6 - LV
7 - SP
8 - KD
9 - SI
10 - TH
11 - KD
12 - LI
13 - BL

Figure 2-8d

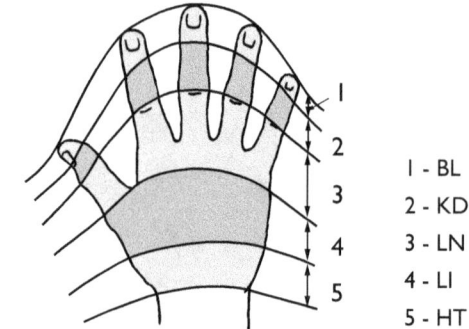

1 - BL
2 - KD
3 - LN
4 - LI
5 - HT

Figure 2-8f

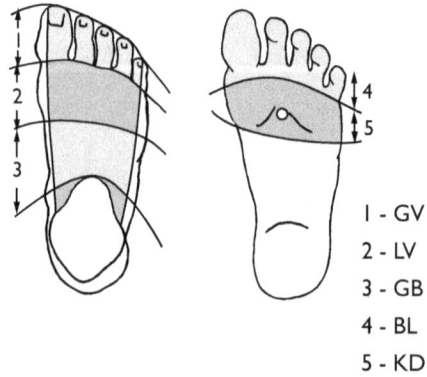

1 - GV
2 - LV
3 - GB
4 - BL
5 - KD

Figure 2-8g

Comparing the Masunaga and Saito Back Charts

I do not believe Masunaga had identified the meridian belt zones as such. However, striking overlaps with his back diagnostic chart (figures 2-9a,b) became apparent as soon as I began charting the belt zones for the back. Only slight discrepancies occur in our respective views of the Triple Heater, Kidney, and Large Intestine meridian zones.

The Link Between Meridian Belt Zones and Meridian Stretch Positions

When following Masunaga's Zen Shiatsu protocol, the patient's leg is bent at the knee at a very particular angle depending on the meridian being treated. I had always wondered how Masunaga determined this: what was he sensing with his *meijin-gei* (master's skill)?

I began studying his leg positions in relation to the meridian belt zones. For example, figure 2-10 on the right illustrates the Liver Meridian stretch positions; on the left, we see the corresponding meridian belt zones, with upper and lower borders clearly demarcated. I found that when you set the patient's heel at the lower border of the Liver Meridian belt zone, the Liver Meridian begins to flow in the pattern of a second-degree imbalance. When you set the patient's heel at the upper border of the belt zone and test for the meridian location, third-degree flow appears (see your *Reference Manual* for an overview of the Regular Meridian pathways).

In subsequent chapters we will learn how to treat meridian imbalances by positioning the patient's legs and arms in these particular ways.

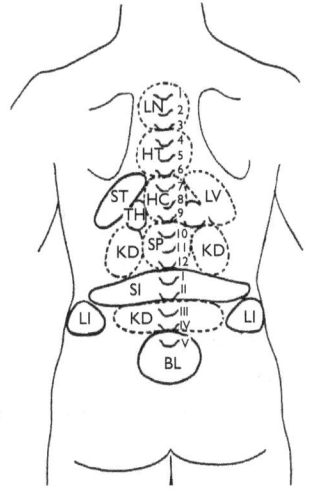

Figure 2-9a Masunaga's back diagnostic chart

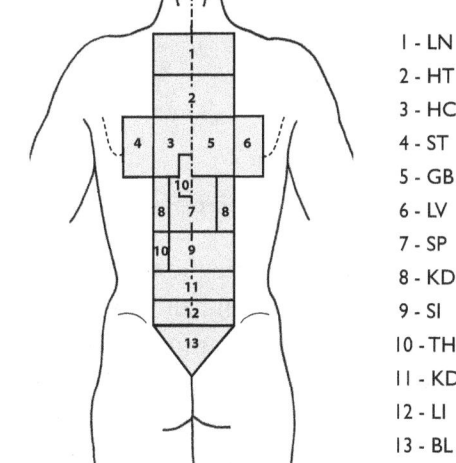

1 - LN
2 - HT
3 - HC
4 - ST
5 - GB
6 - LV
7 - SP
8 - KD
9 - SI
10 - TH
11 - KD
12 - LI
13 - BL

Figure 2-9b Saito's back diagnostic chart

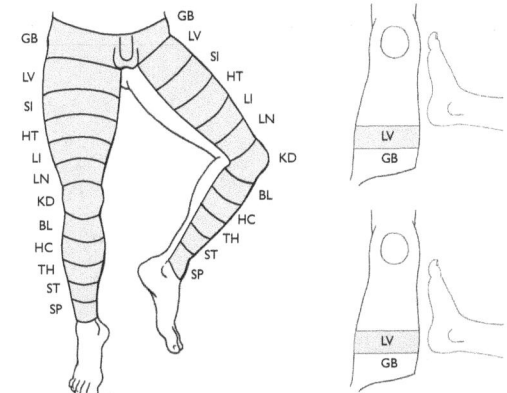

Figure 2-10a
Regular Meridian belt zones

Figure 2-10b
Liver Meridian stretch positions

The Link Between Meridian Belt Zones and Organ Functions

The sequence in which the belt zones occur varies slightly depending on their general location on the body. No matter where they occur, however, yin-yang meridian pairings (Lung/Large Intestine, Spleen/Stomach, Heart/Small Intestine, and so on, as in figure 2-11) remain consistent.

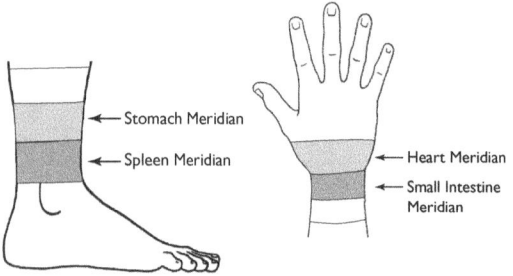

Figure 2-11 Meridian belt zones occur in pairs.

When we examine the sequence of the Regular Meridian belt zones on the arms and legs, another interesting picture emerges: each limb energetically "mirrors" the entire body (figure 2-12). Belt zones on the hand correspond to organ functions of the head, face, and upper chest areas; belt zones on the forearm relate to organ functions of the chest and upper abdomen; belt zones on the upper arm relate to organ functions in the lower abdomen. The bottom of the foot correlates with functions associated with the head and face; the top of the foot is associated with the chest and upper abdominal area; the lower leg correlates with organs in the abdominal area.

This suggests the degree to which our treatment of the arms and legs can affect organ energetics, and points to why so many important acupuncture points on the TCM chart are found distal to the elbow and knees.

Our Intelligent Hands and Feet

Our hands and feet are telling examples of these internal-external links. Very brain-like qualities have been attributed to our fingers: amazing amounts of information about the world around us are deciphered through them. In Japan, it is widely believed that enhancing the sensitivity in our fingers, and especially our fingertips, helps us develop a sharper mind and reduces potential memory loss due to age. This notion extends to the feet and toes. Qi Gong has long incorporated points on the feet and toes to stimulate brain and nerve function via the meridian system. Contemporary science confirms this: studies show how people who walk regularly enjoy better brain function and better all-round health than those who don't.

Attributing brain-like qualities to our hands, fingers, feet, and toes, makes more sense when we look at meridian routes and belt zones. Belt zones for the Kidney and Bladder are found at the fingertips and under the toes (see figures 2-8f and 2-8g). It has been found that when people lose the use of their hands, they tend to enhance the use of their feet. Essentially, they are

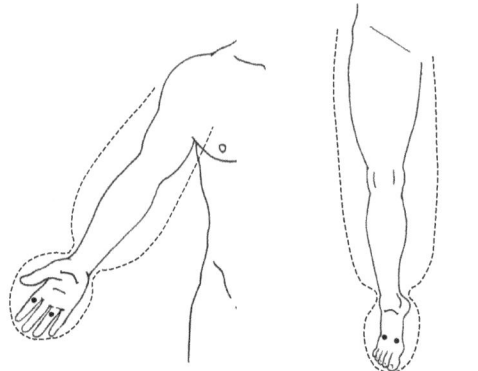

Figure 2-12 Meridian belt zones mirror the body.

fine-tuning their sensitivity here, where the Kidney and Bladder meridian belt zones are located. Masunaga also observed how the Kidney and Bladder meridians governed brain and nerve function.

The Hirata Zones

Although relatively unknown in the West, Kurakichi Hirata (1901-1945) has been one of modern Japan's most influential researchers and practitioners in the field of Oriental medicine. He began his academic career studying philosophy and psychology at Kyoto University before undertaking a degree in Western medicine. After being introduced to the Oriental approach, however, he abandoned his Western medical studies to explore various branches of Chinese medicine, including acupuncture, meridian shiatsu, and exercise. I find it noteworthy that Hirata did not restrict his research to the professional elite, but made his work accessible to the general public, so that it could be used for the purposes of preventative medicine. His achievements included his discovery of the Hirata Zones (figure 2.5) — 12 numbered zones, appearing sequentially on the head, neck, trunk, arms and legs, and each relating to a specific organ.

Hirata greatly influenced Masunaga (1925-1981), who would also become a distinguished practitioner in the realm of Oriental medicine. Interestingly, both men attended the same university and began their pursuits with a foundation in the study of psychology.

More than half a century has passed since Hirata presented us with his chart, a source of inspiration and intrigue for me. I was most curious to know if there was a link between Hirata's zones and meridian energetics.

The mystery was solved as I undertook to draw the belt zones for Divergent Meridians (Chapter 7), and saw Hirata's pattern emerging before my eyes. In my completed chart were the belt zones for the Divergent Meridians — an extension of the Regular Meridian system —which carry ki from the body's surface to the organs. In Hirata's chart, we see, simply, "belt zones" for the organs. Two charts with different names and labels, telling the same story.

Here are more interesting similarities and differences in our work:

- The Hirata Zones link the fingers and toes to the genital organs; my chart of the Divergent Meridian belt zones links the genital organs to the Governor and Conception meridians, part of the Extra Meridian system. My work on the Extra Meridian system strongly links these two Extra Meridians to the Liver and Gallbladder meridians. The Liver and Gallbladder meridians are also closely related to the genital organs: the TCM chart shows the Liver Meridian flowing into the genital organs.

- The Hirata Zones show no correlates for either the Triple Heater and Heart Constrictor meridians, which do appear in my Divergent Meridian belt zones.

- For any level of imbalance (first, second, or third degree) the sequence of Regular Meridian belt zones on the forearm closely parallels the locations of these organs in the abdominal area. See figure 2-12. When the Divergent Meridian system is engaged, the belt zones on the upper arm parallel Hirata's zones. This order is reversed on the leg (figure 2-13).

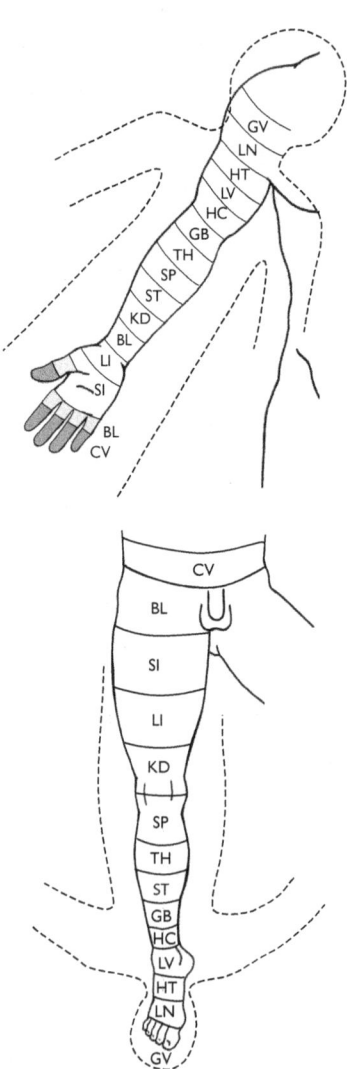

Much remains to be learned about meridian belt zones. What I know about them so far has been integral to my development of the Shin So Shiatsu system. Before he died, Dr. Tadashi Irie expressed great interest in what he called my "revolutionary discovery," suggesting it would have an enormous impact on meridian-energetics theory. The challenge ahead is to further develop this phenomenon's potential as a diagnostic and treatment tool.

Figure 2-13 Divergent Meridian belt zones parallel Hirata's zones.

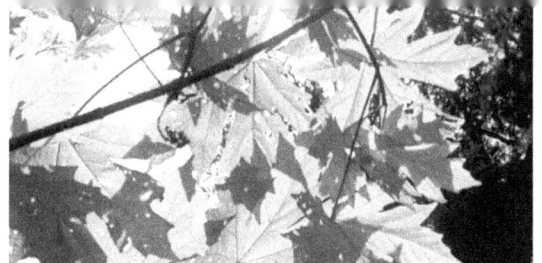

3
Sensing Energy

quiet —
in the depths of the lake
a peak of cloud

- Issa Kobayashi -

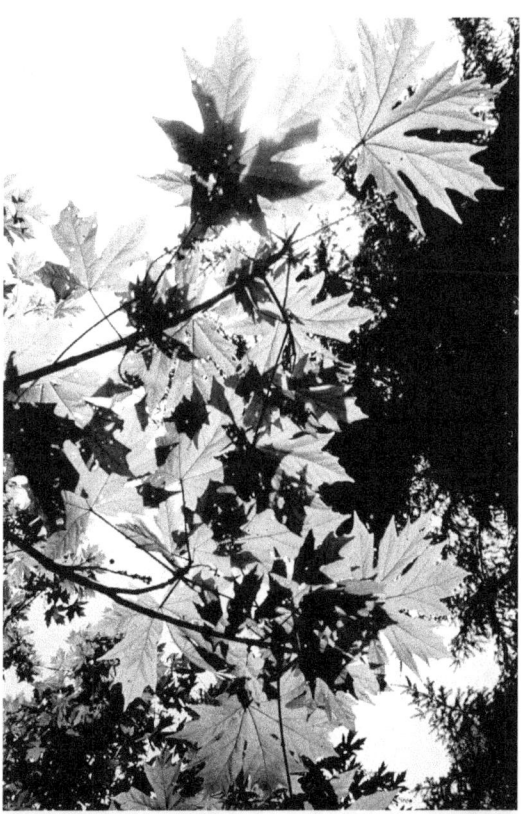

In this chapter, you will learn:

- How to prepare yourself and your patients for work with the finger test.

- How to perform the finger test.

- How to finger test foods and supplements.

- How to use the finger test and sound imaging to locate specific body structures.

- How to trace Regular Meridians using the finger test.

Chapter 3

Sensing Energy

This chapter takes us from theory to practice. From the potentially confusing array of maps, charts, and line drawings that describe meridians and other energetic phenomena, to the actual experience of finding them, feeling them, and following them around the body.

This chapter is about how we can increase our sensitivity to the ki-meridian system. How we can learn to "speak" ki — literally talk to the meridians using the language of the Finger Test Method. We are asking them questions, hearing their answers. And then, going further, guiding the meridians with our intentions, touching them with our hands and our hearts, supporting their imperative to achieve balance.

Though imperceptible to most people, ki is a substance. Its responsiveness to frequency, vibration, and pressure is what underlies our work as practitioners of Oriental medicine. In contrast to modern medical specialists who rely on highly technical equipment to diagnose their patients, practitioners of Oriental medicine must develop in their own bodies a fine sensitivity to the subtleties of ki. Potentially, this can provide us with nearly everything we need to know about what is happening in the patient's body.

Listen with your Tanden

In many Eastern traditions, training focuses on the tanden, located just below the navel. Attunement with this powerful energy core deepens our responsiveness to the rarefied vibrational aspect of ki. The subtle and mesmerizing beauty of a well-tended Zen garden, the simplicity of the Japanese tea ceremony, or a well-executed kata in martial arts are all expressions of the smooth and harmonious flow of ki through the artist. Likewise, the ability to heal others flows from the tanden.

Shizuto Masunaga continually encouraged us to turn off our busy minds and "listen" with our tandens. Only in this way, he said, can we understand what the body is telling us at this very instant. And it is to the body's condition, in this instant, that our treatment must respond.

Our daily shiatsu practice is one of the

many ways we can develop our tandens: maintaining correct posture, deep breathing, and a calm mind will bring strength to this important energy centre. Meditation, qi gong, tai chi, and yoga are other helpful disciplines.

A good grounding in the broader concept of the ki-meridian system deepens our understanding of the nature and behavior of energy and how it infuses us with spirit and vitality. Our state of health is reflected in the flow and patterning of ki throughout our bodies. With the onset of disease, from either external or internal causes, we see the ki-meridian system in action as it sets out to eliminate it, even to the point that individual meridians exhaust themselves. For all of these patterns and tendencies, we have names and categories — meridian systems, levels of imbalance, qualities of imbalance (such as kyo and jitsu) — that serve as powerful diagnostic tools.

Without this ki-meridian system — this vast geography with its many benchmarks, milestones, and landmarks — it would not only be difficult for us to know where we are now (diagnosis). It would be difficult for us to know where we might like to go (treatment). Central to working with the ki-meridian system is our ability to imagine, or "image." From this comes our ability to form intention. The ancient Chinese spoke of this as *yi*, or thought. The adage "ki follows *yi* and blood follows ki" describes how the classics viewed the role of intention in treatments. With a clear map of the terrain ahead it is far easier to form a strong intention about treatment outcome, and this makes arriving at our destination more straightforward. In other words, our shiatsu treatments will be more precise and appropriate.

Dr. Tadashi Irie
Inventor of the Finger Test Method

Dr. Tadashi Irie, highly regarded in Japan for his research in the field of acupuncture, developed the Irie finger test technique in the 1980s. From the outset, it was a useful tool in determining point locations, but his main purpose was to find an alternative to pulse diagnosis, which takes years of practice to master. Discovering that the finger test could be learned quickly and used accurately and efficiently, he went on to develop a comprehensive diagnostic system and treatment protocols for balancing the Extra, Divergent, and Muscle meridians.

It was about this time that I began my own search for a practical alternative to Shizuto Masunaga's hara diagnostic system. While I appreciated Masunaga's groundbreaking insights, I had come to realize that practitioners would have to possess his sensitivity to energy flows in order to accurately use his diagnostic methods. Chancing upon Dr. Irie's Finger Test Method, I began a lifetime of intensive exploration with it.

Dr. Irie passed away in 2002. Today in Japan, his Finger Test Method is widely known, and many acupuncturists use it. Meanwhile, researchers continue to explore its applications.

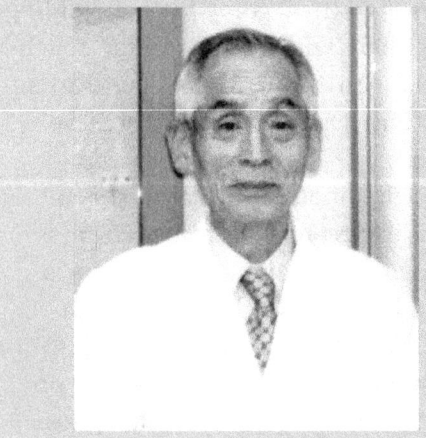

Figure 3-1 Dr. Tadashi Irie

Performing the Finger Test
What Are You Looking for?

When using the finger test to diagnose the ki-meridian system, it is essential that we maintain a clear image of what it is we are looking for. What energy systems are we evaluating, which meridians are we evaluating, and are they kyo or jitsu in nature? In time, we will learn to tune into these different channels of the body just as we tune into radio stations, first by selecting the frequency (the image) and then by using the antenna (the sensor) to locate the image and bring it into focus.

Without a clear image of the meridians or diagnostic zones we are trying to locate or treat, it is as if we are playing with the radio dial. The result will be the same: we will pick up a lot of static or confused energy, and find ourselves unable get a clear picture of the patient's condition. Practice and familiarity are paramount to achieving success with this technique.

How the Finger Test Method Works

The Finger Test Method works much like a television set. The antenna receives a multitude of waves or signals from one or several transmitting stations. These are delivered to the tuner, where one wave (channel) is selected. This is amplified and sent to the television screen, where the selected program can be viewed. Figure 3-2 illustrates this.

The meridian system stores, receives, and sends out information about the human body. Our hands are especially important in their capacity to project energetic information into the environment and retrieve it. In our television analogy, one hand serves as the antenna — or what

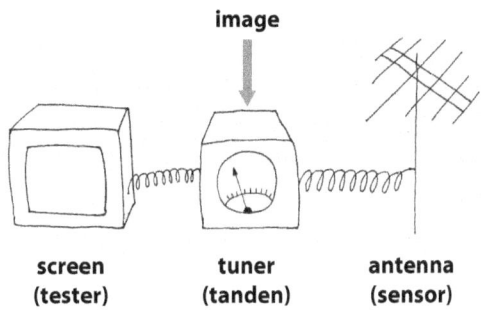

Figure 3-2 The finger test works like a TV set.

we call the sensor — which receives information. The other hand is the tester, like a television screen in that it displays the answer we are looking for.

Once we have received an energy transmission, the information travels from the sensor, by way of our own meridian system, to our tanden. Here, we must tune in, or select the particular information that we are searching for. It is imperative to maintain a very clear image of the energies we are diagnosing. In other words, what do we want to know? We want our tester to respond only to this question and not anything else from the barrage of noise constantly swirling about us. I must emphasize here, too, how important it is that our information request be sent to the tanden (or tuner) and not to the busy mind. A vague or distorted question will get a vague or distorted answer. Masunaga knew this too, and taught us to keep our minds at rest, or in a meditative state, when diagnosing the meridian system. This is how his approach became distinguished as Zen Shiatsu.

Our Hands are Sensors

Based on a deep appreciation of the responsiveness of the human hand and its capacity to send and receive energy, Eastern meditative traditions have identified certain hand positions or mudras that help us communicate with the energy around and within us. There are 12 main Shin So sensors, each with its own purpose, as shown in your *Reference Manual*. Most of these have been developed through years of research, through trial and error in my own practice and the occasional gift of pure inspiration. Three in particular (the ja ki, chakra, virus/parasite sensors) were first identified by Dr. Hideo Yoshimoto.

The finger test is similar in many ways to the O-Ring Test and other versions of applied kinesiology and muscle testing. The main difference is that we can perform the finger test easily ourselves — with one hand. This leaves the other hand free to form the Shin So sensors, greatly enhancing the range of information we can derive. The benefits that come from developing our sensitivity through practice with these sensors cannot be overstated.

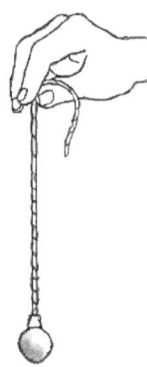

Figure 3-3 Our hands are extremely sensitive. Each finger emits a specific bioenergetic charge. Those experienced with pendulums will be familiar with this. A pendulum will swing in a clockwise direction when gently held over the index and ring fingers. When held over the middle or little fingers, it will swing the other way. When held over the thumb, a pendulum generally swings back and forth, denoting a neutral charge.

Instruction
Preparing to perform the finger test

1. Remove all jewelry, watches, gems, medicines or other possible sources of interference from yourself and your patient.

2. Remove strong magnetic fields from the treatment area.

3. Clear surface ja ki from yourself and your patient (see "clearing surface ja ki," below).

4. The first of these steps may be omitted once we have a sufficient mastery of the Finger Test Method and a well-developed tanden. Regardless of our level of experience, however, it is still wise to avoid the electromagnetic interference of radios, televisions, computers, fans, and other appliances. And it is always necessary to remove ja ki from around both the therapist and the patient. Ja ki interferes with this style of diagnosis and can easily cause misdiagnosis.

Instruction
Performing the finger test

Developing accuracy and confidence with the Finger Test Method requires daily practice. We are in effect learning a new language.

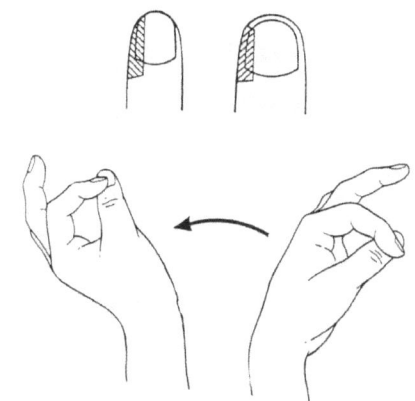

Figure 3-4 Overlap the index finger and thumb and slowly slide the thumb over the edge of the index finger like a bow moving over a violin.

1. First, relax your wrist and shoulder. Overlap your thumb and index finger, as indicated in figure 3-4, and slide your thumb slowly over the index finger. Either hand can be used for this purpose: this is your tester hand. The other will be your "sensor" hand. Whether you are diagnosing the ki-meridian system or testing food and supplements (see below), there are only two sensations your tester hand can register: sticky or smooth. Stickiness feels as if there is a bit of glue or dewy moisture between your index finger and thumb. Smoothness is when the fingers can slide unimpeded.

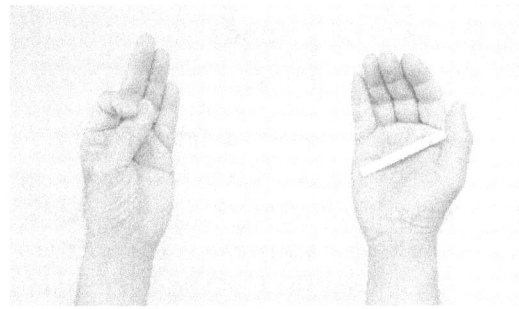

Figure 3-5 Practicing the finger test with powerful substances like cigarettes teaches us how to read our strongest energetic responses.

2. Try this experiment. Place a cigarette in the palm of your sensor hand and very slowly operate the tester (i.e. rub together index finger and thumb). The image you might project to your tanden is actually a question: is this cigarette good for your system? Most people will feel a change in the tester hand — a stickiness where the index finger rubs over the thumb. This means the answer to your question is no. Smoothness, or no change in the sensation between the two fingers, means the answer is yes.

Finger Testing Foods and Supplements

Just as the Finger Test Method can be used to locate meridians, identify meridians that are out of balance, and diagnose a multitude of conditions, it can also be used to diagnose our body's energetic responses to foods, drinks, and supplements (vitamins and pharmaceuticals). Commonly finger-tested items include wheat, dairy, sugar, and caffeine products: if you can eat it, you can test it.

> **Instruction**
> **Finger testing foods and supplements**
>
> 1. Prepare products for finger testing. Remove any aluminum foil wrappings. If testing fruit, such as bananas or oranges, image the edible portion (i.e. imagine the fruit without its skin). If a supplement or medicine is inside a capsule, you will need to image the contents and the capsule separately: some people react to the capsules. Place small food items to be tested in the palm of your right (or sensor) hand; put larger items on a plate and position your sensor hand over the product. Pour drinks into cups and direct your pointer finger toward the contents.
>
> 2. Image for quantity. For example, if you are holding a bottle of 100 tablets, you might first image the question, "does one capsule agree with my system?" Then, image whether two, three, four tablets, and so on, agree with your system. Likewise, with other substances, you can image for quantity: half a cup, or a whole cup?
>
> 3. Follow the procedure outlined under "Performing the finger test" for diagnosing your body's response to a cigarette.

Now Add Sound Imaging

In scanning the patient's body with open hands we may pick up heat or cold, wind-like sensations, or a tingling associated with areas where energy is flowing too quickly or in excess. By combining sound imaging with the finger test, we obtain even more information from the body's vibrations. There are sound images to help us identify each vertebra of the spine, each meridian system, meridian, and meridian diagnostic zone. Others help us to find problems with specific joints, bacterial or viral infections, and dental issues. There is even a sound image to help us locate the presence of ja ki, or "negative energy" in the body (see below).

Japanese doctors, Hajime Oda, M.D. (*Ki and Ki Diagnosis*, Shinkyu Kishin Kenkyu Kai, 1996) and Masaaki Suehara, Ph.D, D.C. (*Onsho Shindan Gaku*, 1984, and *Gen So Keiraku Ho*, 1985, Onsho Shindan Gaku Kenkyu Sho) have investigated how sound and sound imaging affect the human energy system. They suggest certain sound vibrations (including inaudible sound images) trigger a response — actually a weakness — in the muscles, bones, and meridian systems. In other words, certain sound images act as "off switches" for certain meridians or structures. For example, in the practice of Shin So Shiatsu, we image the sound that correlates to a particular meridian or body structure, and when our sensor encounters that structure, we experience a sticky sensation. The sound image's vibrations temporarily interrupt the natural harmonics of the structure we are looking for, and the finger test's sticky sensation is a response to that.

Shin So Shiatsu uses many sound images: they are provided in your *Reference Manual*.

Dealing with Surface Ja ki

Ja ki — energy that interferes with the flow of sei ki (our good or healthy energy) — can be found both on the body's surface and deeper within our energy system. In the practice of Shin So Shiatsu, the main problem with surface ja ki is its interference with energy diagnosis. It may create the appearance of a completely new energy flow (mimicking third-degree flow), or cause segments of normal energy flow to disappear temporarily. To avoid distorted readings, it is essential to follow the procedure outlined here for removing this particular form of ja ki. Deeper-level ja ki is discussed in Chapter 4.

Dr. Hajime Oda cites two common sources for the ja ki we find on the body's surface as well as at deeper levels within the body. One is the electromagnetic field created by any number of appliances we encounter in our daily lives (televisions, computers, fans). Scientists are just beginning to report the significant health hazards associated with the more powerful sources of electromagnetic energy, such as high voltage wires.

The second most common source of surface ja ki is people. Energy relates to energy at a vibrational level, and ja ki radiating from one person may attach itself to others. Energy is released in quantity in therapeutic environments, and practitioners have been known to experience ja ki in the form of headaches, fatigue or malaise. The impact of ja ki in this setting tends to be minimal, depending on the condition of both the therapist and his or her patients. Therapists who frequently treat patients with serious illnesses will need to be more attuned to its effects.

I nevertheless strongly recommend we incorporate ja ki removal into our daily lives through such simple practices as hand washing, meditation, or techniques such as the following.

Finger Test-imonials

"In shiatsu, we are meant to be working with energy, but until I learned the Finger Test Method, I couldn't sense its flow. I didn't know exactly where the meridians were."
— Marthy Dehntroven, Switzerland

"Incorporating the Finger Test Method into my shiatsu treatments — as well as the rest of my life — has been the greatest benefit of any training I have ever done. Diagnosis used to be the most difficult aspect of my work. Now my treatments are very precise, meeting the patient's needs. My confidence has blossomed."
— Ursula Kroer, Austria

"The finger test has helped deepen my understanding of the body's healing processes and turned my treatments into light and playful work."
— Jaya Doris Huggler, Switzerland

Instruction
Clearing surface ja ki

This type of ja ki accumulates progressively from feet upward to the head, as shown in figure 3-6.

1. Move your sensor hand slowly toward the patient's feet, and image the sound "A-o." The palm of your sensor hand should be fully open and facing the patient's feet. If ja ki is present, the tester hand will read sticky as soon as your sensor hand meets the upper edge of this energy accumulation. See figure 3-7a.

2. Having confirmed the presence of ja ki, you must now image and locate the two "holes" used in the process of flushing it from the body. A black hole lies somewhere on the centre line of the upper body, a white hole lies along the centre line of one of the legs. Image the black hole first, while sweeping your hand in the general sensor position from the top of the patient's head downward along the Conception Vessel. The tester hand will read sticky when your sensor hand encounters the black hole. Now, scan the patient's lower body for the white hole (figure 3-7b).

3. Place your hands gently above the two holes, and send energy simultaneously into both (as though to allow our projected ki to get beneath the ja ki) with the aim of pushing the accumulated ja ki up and away from the patient's body. Ja ki is unstable, and easily influenced by other vibrating energies (figure 3-7c).

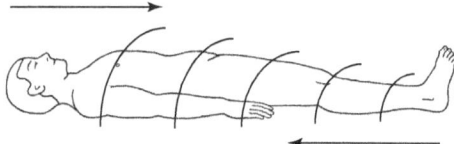

Figure 3-6 Ja ki covers us from the feet upwards.

4. Now that the ja ki has been pushed up, re-circulate the patient's ki. Making a small circular motion with your hand, 15 to 20 times, encourages their ki to circulate up the back of their body via the Governing Vessel, and then down the front of their body via the Conception Vessel (figure 3-7d).

5. Check for any remaining ja ki by repeating Step 1. If the finger test reads sticky at any point as you re-scan the patient from head to foot, repeat steps 2-4. Residual ja ki may continue to hover just above the surface of the body. To check for this, place your sensor hand palm up (away from the patient's body), and again image the sound "A-o" (figure 3-7e). If the finger test still proves sticky, go to step 6.

6. Face your patient, place your hands together at the palms, in the energetically potent gesture of prayer (called *ga sho* in Japanese) and simply ask for the ja ki to leave (figure 3-7f). It is now possible to accurately diagnose and locate the meridian pathways.

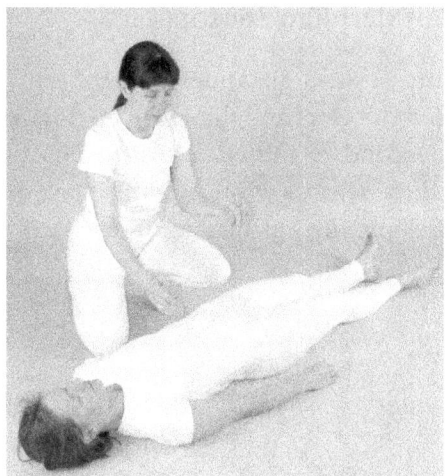
Figure 3-7a Scan for ja ki.

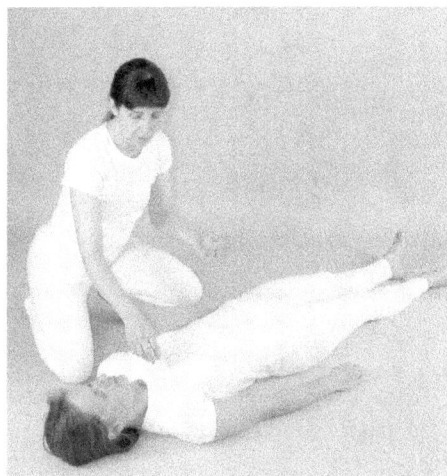
Figure 3-7b Locate two energy holes.

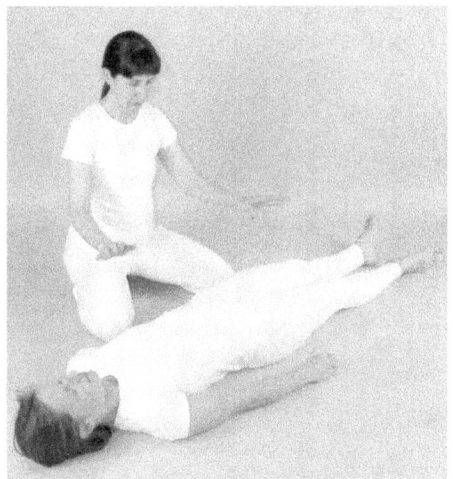
Figure 3-7c Send energy into body.

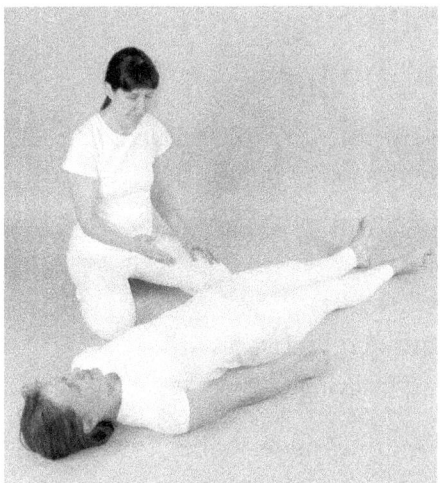
Figure 3-7d Circulate ki.

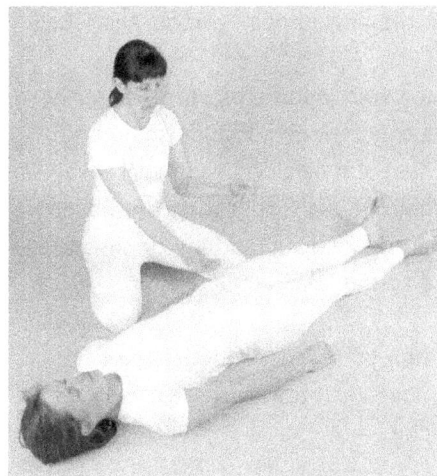
Figure 3-7e Check for residual ja ki.

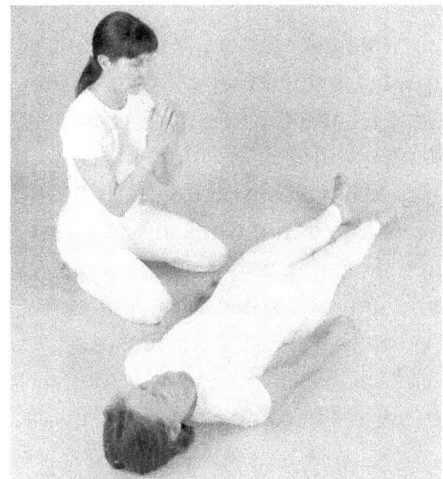
Figure 3-7f Ask residual ja ki to leave.

More Practice with Sound Images

Once again, refer to your *Reference Manual*, and note the sound images that can be used to locate specific vertebrae.

> **Instruction**
> Locating vertebrae with sound imaging
>
> 1. In your *Reference Manual*, look for the sound correlate for the vertebra you wish to find. For example, the sound for the first lumbar vertebra is "Ba."
>
> 2. Place your middle or index finger at the top of your patient's spine and glide it slowly along each vertebra, simultaneously operating the finger test and imaging (audibly or silently) the sound "Ba."
>
> 3. When your sensor meets the first lumbar vertebra, the tester will feel sticky.

Sensing Meridians

Practicing the finger test with foods and substances has helped prepare you for the task of sensing and tracing meridians. As my students around the world will tell you, this is easier than you might think. But don't be lulled into thinking no effort is required. Locating and tracing meridians and their diagnostic zones takes practice: in this, we are developing our sensitivity and enhancing our ki level. I strongly recommend this become a regular exercise.

Regular Meridian Sensors

Figures 3-8a, 3-8b, and 3-8c show sensors used to detect and diagnose meridians at first, second, or third degree imbalance. Using these sensors while holding a pen or chopstick provides greater accuracy.

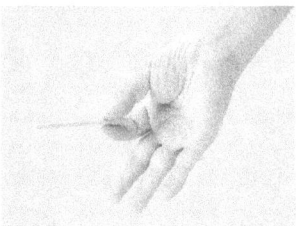

Figure 3-8a First-degree sensor

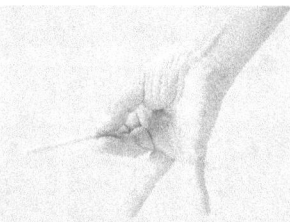

Figure 3-8b Second-degree sensor

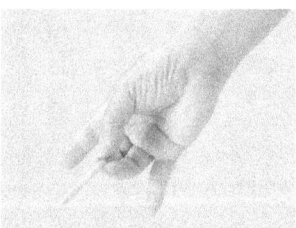

Figure 3-8c Third-degree sensor

Instruction
Sensing Regular Meridians

1. Clear surface ja ki from therapist and patient.

2. Choose the appropriate sensor. The sensor most commonly used in meridian location is the general sensor, formed using the three middle fingers (index, middle, and ring fingers) held closely together as in figure 3-9. Figure 3-10 illustrates how a pointed object such as a pen or chopstick held with your fingers in the same sensing position enhances precision for purposes of diagnosis or research.

3. Image the name of the meridian you are looking for. Your sensor will pick up the specific pathway in which the ki is currently vibrating — first, second, or third degree. As an alternative to imaging the meridian name, you can image the sound associated with the meridian you are looking for. However, in this case, your sensor will pick up all of the pathways associated with that meridian, whether they are vibrating or not.

4. Begin finger testing. Slide your sensor (or sensor and chopstick) slowly toward the meridian pathway. When the sensor meets the meridian you are looking for, your tester will feel sticky.

5. Figures 3-9 and 3-11 show the meridian as a thin line. As I explained in Chapter 1, Regular Meridians are actually much wider. To feel this width for yourself, move your sensor toward the meridian from both sides of its pathway, as in figure 3-11. When your tester crosses the outer edges of the pathway, your tester will feel sticky.

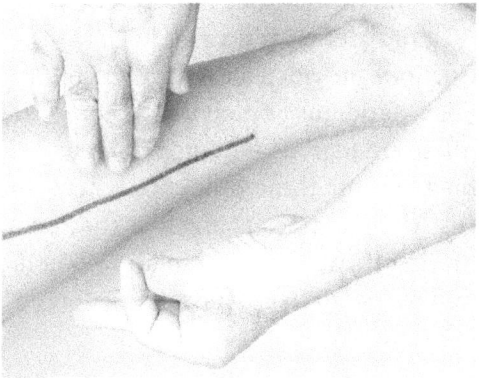

Figure 3-9 Tracing Regular Meridians with the general sensor

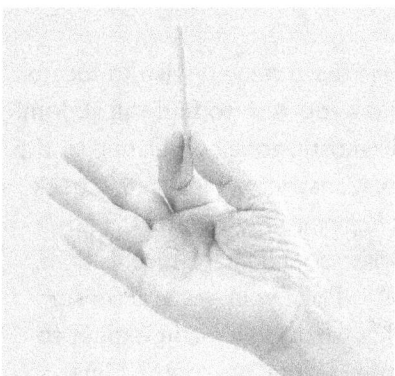

Figure 3-10

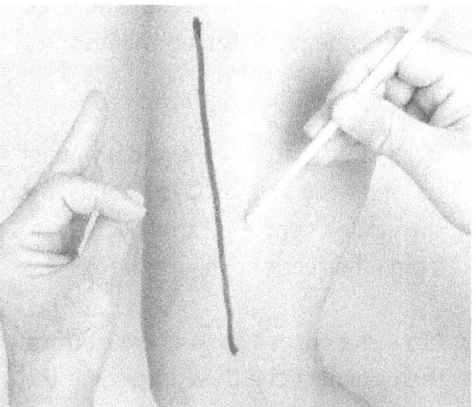

Figure 3-11 Sensing with a chopstick increases accuracy.

Sensing Abdominal Diagnostic Zones

Abdominal diagnostic zones are an important and useful manifestation of first, second, and third degree imbalances in the Regular Meridian system. Review the instructions provided above for sensing Regular Meridians as preparation for locating these circular areas. Once you have learned to sense these zones accurately you can use them to track changes as they occur during treatments, and to know when a given meridian needs more work.

Instruction

Sensing abdominal diagnostic zones

1. Choose the zone you wish to locate. Let's say you wish to find the abdominal diagnostic zone correlating to the Heart Constrictor Meridian. Check your *Reference Manual* for the appropriate sound image (in this case, "Gyo"). Place your general sensor roughly where you might expect to find the Heart Constrictor Meridian zone, and image the sound "Gyo." When your sensor reaches the edge of the zone, your tester will feel sticky.

2. Using a washable pen and continuing to image the sound "Gyo," focus in on the circle's centre by approaching it from all directions (figure 3-13).

3. Mark the edges with a circle of dots, then connect the dots to outline the zone (figure 3-14).

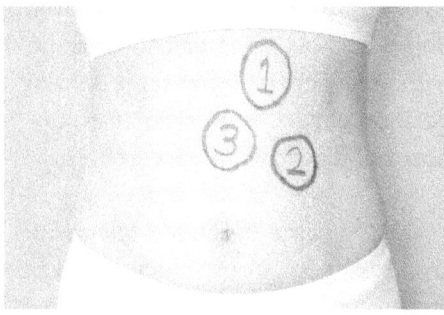

Figure 3-12 First-, second-, and third-degree diagnostic zones for the Stomach Meridian

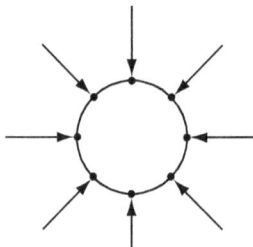

Figure 3-13 Approach energy circles from the outside in

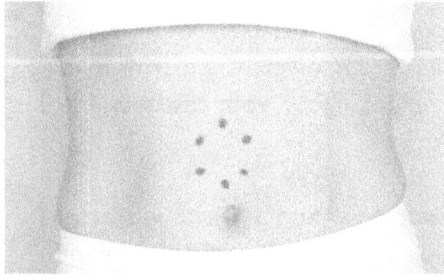

Figure 3-14 Tracing the first-degree Heart Constrictor diagnostic zone

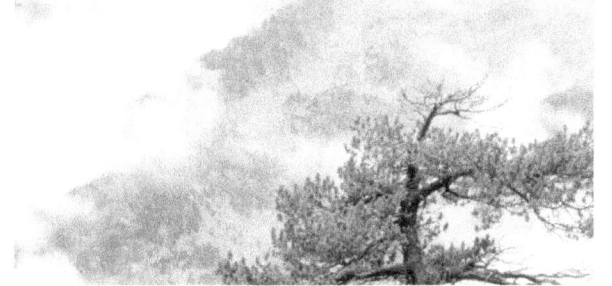

4

Shin So Shiatsu
Goals and Methods

a new year
rain-catching stone
about to burst

- Issa Kobayashi -

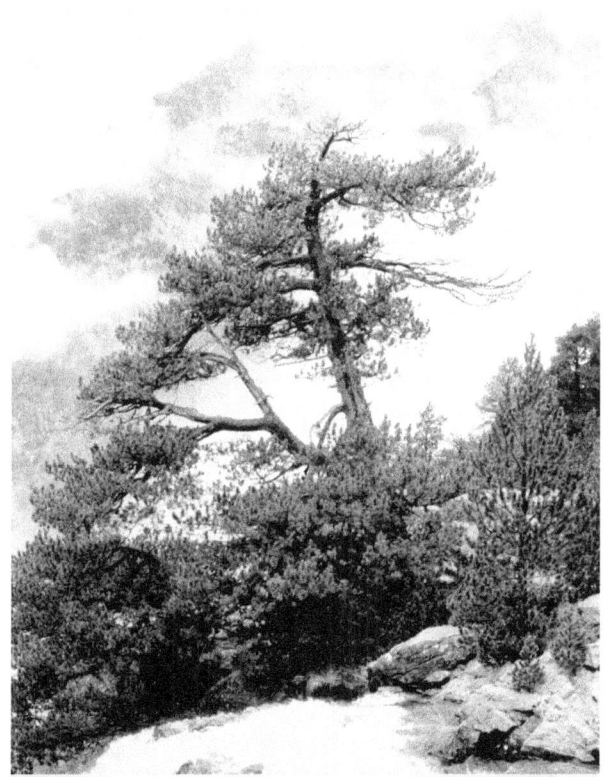

In this chapter, you will learn:

- How to diagnose the deepest level of meridian imbalance.

- How to diagnose structural problems.

- How to treat structural problems with diodes.

- How to seal off sources of ja ki in a room.

- How to prepare for possible treatment responses.

Chapter 4

Shin So Shiatsu
Goals and Methods

You are already sensing and tracing Regular Meridians and energy circles and will soon be prepared for the more advanced work of diagnosing and treating the deeper meridian systems (chapters 5-10). To further prepare you, the basic goals and methods of Shin So Shiatsu and some techniques you will need to get started in any treatment are outlined in this chapter.

Our overview of Shin So Shiatsu's underlying principles begins with a closer look at ki, or more specifically, the dynamic relationship between sei ki and ja ki that is so central to our approach.

About Sei ki and Ja ki

There are two kinds of ki. We are most familiar with sei ki — our "pure" or "healthy" energy as it is derived from three sources: our parents (i.e. our genetic inheritance), cosmic energy, and the food and water we ingest. Sei ki flows throughout our bodies via the meridian systems: it protects us from disease, supports us, keeps us healthy.

Ja ki — often translated into English as "negative energy," is energy that interferes with the flow of sei ki. Shizuto Masunaga translated ja to mean "what happens when gears don't mesh properly." He taught us simply that ja ki is a form of energy that does not co-exist harmoniously with sei ki. Ja ki can be found at two general locations. In Chapter 3, we learned to sense and eliminate ja ki from the body's surface, where its presence creates unusual vibrational terrains and interferes with our ability to diagnose the meridian systems. Ja ki also manifests deeper within the body. TCM says ja ki creates jitsu-like conditions at these deeper levels. In other words, it manifests as patient-felt symptoms. Links between surface ja ki and internal ja ki remain to be explored.

Although TCM acknowledges internal ja ki, it has been the focus of relatively little attention from either the acupuncture or shiatsu professions. My research has convinced me how integral ja ki is to human energetics. I have found that in the most serious cases of illness, not only are the meridians out of balance, but ja ki is also implicated. I have also seen that while eliminating ja ki can actually balance sei ki in the meridians, addressing the deepest meridian imbalances may not have any impact on ja ki. This suggests to me that, especially in the most serious cases, ja ki is the deeper source of the problem.

How Internal Ja ki is Created

Meikan Okudaira, in his book, *Ja-ki Ron* (Ido No Nippon Sha, 1999), suggests ja ki is created when our sei ki tries to expel bodily intruders. Take this simple example. Your own natural healing energy undertakes to eliminate a virus. Here we have the two gears that Masunaga describes as not meshing well: one is sei ki, the other is the virus, and now, as a result of their encounter — there is ja ki.

Okudaira divides bodily invaders into the following categories:

1. Intruders from outside the body
   (as described in TCM texts).
   a. Wind b. Heat c. Damp d. Dry e. Cold
   Other intruders include viruses, bacteria, parasites, radiation, magnetic fields.

2. Strong emotions
   (also described in TCM texts).
   a. Anger b. Fear c. Worry d. Grief
   e. Joy

3. A combination of intruders from outside the body and strong emotions.

I believe there are many other ways internal ja ki is generated and that further research will shed more light on this and ways to reduce their impact. I also believe, however, that ja ki can never be completely eliminated from our bodies: that it will, to some degree, always be with us. In fact, it is proof we are alive. Even when our sei ki is technically "in balance," some degree of imbalance always remains (see Chapter 1). And just as ja ki is proof we are alive, so are these minor imbalances.

I see the accumulation of ja ki in the body as being like the buildup of sediment on a riverbottom, where it eventually interferes with the river's flow (figure 4-1). Rocks, boulders, branches, and stumps get caught up in it, and create a bigger blockage. Like muscular tension along the energy pathways, this degree of buildup is easily detected through touch. But just as the initial accumulation of sediment under moving water is hard to detect, so is ja ki, at first deeply hidden, though already creating problems. Removing it from beneath the water flow may require repeated attempts, and we may even consider the intervention of powerful machinery. In the process of such a clean up, the river itself may hamper our efforts, creating more problems.

Shin So Shiatsu takes a practical approach, seeking both to regulate sei ki imbalances and to eliminate as much ja ki from our bodies as possible.

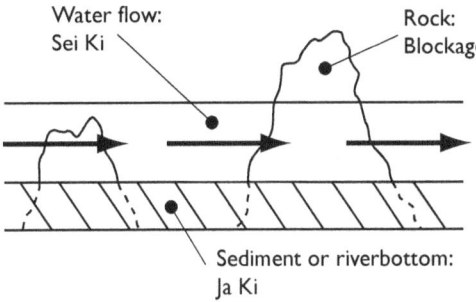

Figure 4-1 Ja ki accumulates in our bodies much in the same way as sediment builds up on a riverbottom.

The Three Main Goals of Shin So Shiatsu

How we approach each of these will vary case by case, but we should not ignore any of them:

1. Balancing sei ki

Using Shin So Shiatsu's treatment methods, we can achieve balance in the meridians. But for how long? A second, a minute, or more? The longer our sei ki is in balance, the more opportunity the body has to heal itself. When the patient's condition is not very serious (and a minimum of ja ki has accumulated), we emphasize this treatment goal. For example, if we are addressing what is mainly a structural problem, we would perform a yaki hari treatment of energy circles resulting from both that structural problem and what we diagnose to be the imbalanced meridian system. This addresses the patient's "problem area" and the sei ki imbalance, and there is no need for further treatment to remove ja ki.

2. Eliminating ja ki

Once a patient's condition becomes more serious, with symptoms of mental/emotional or organ dysfunction, we know internal ja ki has begun to accumulate. If we only balance sei ki, the underlying ja ki will push the meridians out of balance again. Conversely, if we eliminate the ja ki, the meridians will respond by re-balancing themselves. This is like clearing sediment from the riverbottom: the river will begin to flow freely itself.

3. Removing meridian blockages

Whether we balance sei ki, eliminate ja ki, or both, a certain amount of muscle tension remains along the meridian pathways. This must be removed to ensure the meridians stay balanced for as long as possible. While this creates a more effective treatment, the degree and focus of this work will vary case by case.

The Two Main Components of a Shin So Treatment

1. Honji treatment

Start with the foundation. Address the deepest level of imbalance first.
In Japanese, *hon* means "basic" or "foundation," and *ji* means "treatment." Our purpose is akin to building a solid foundation for a house. In addressing the

deepest level of imbalance, we support all of the body's energy systems. This increases the patient's overall vitality and prepares them for further treatment (i.e. hyoji treatment).

2. **Hyoji treatment**
   After you stabilize the foundation, address the patient's symptoms.
   Hyoji means "target treatment." In constructing a house, this means focussing on the details. If the patient's symptoms are mainly structural in nature, the main focus of your hyoji treatment will be on balancing sei ki and removing meridian blockages. If the problem is mainly emotional/internal, your focus will be on clearing ja ki and removing meridian blockages.

We will meet the terms honji and hyoji again in our work with the individual meridian systems.

The Four Main Shin So Shiatsu Treatment Methods

To accomplish its honji treatment goals (and in some cases also hyoji treatment goals), Shin So Shiatsu mainly employs the four methods briefly described below. They are covered later in more detail. Which one you use depends on the meridian system you are addressing, your patient's needs, and your own inclinations as a therapist.

1. **Meridian shiatsu**
   Depending on our diagnosis, the Shin So Shiatsu therapist positions their patient with their arms and legs "stretched" in a very particular way, as discussed in Chapter 2. These positions are described in the following chapters and detailed in the *Reference Manual*.

2. **Ja ki clearing**
   While the Chinese have long noted the phenomenon of ja ki in the human body, Japanese practitioners have placed a greater emphasis on finding theoretical and practical approaches for dealing with it. A few centuries ago (we don't know exactly when), a little-known Buddhist monk named Mu Bun Sai studied the links between ja ki and the meridians: the diagnostic charts he devised are an invaluable legacy. In Shin So Shiatsu we use them as a treatment tool for eliminating ja ki (see chapters 6, 7, and 8).

3. **Yaki hari treatment**
   It means "heated needle" in Japanese and was first developed by Kurakichi Hirata and later modified by Dr. Tadashi Irie. In Shin So Shiatsu, a heated metal rod is used to treat energy circles that appear when the Extra and Divergent meridian systems are out of balance, as well as energy circles associated with structural imbalances. This method is detailed in Chapter 6.

4. **Ion pumping**
   This technique, which balances positive and negative ions inside and outside the meridians, will be familiar to acupuncturists. Shin So Shiatsu employs ion-pumping (IP) cords to treat the Extra and Divergent meridian systems in particular. It is detailed in Chapter 6.

Diagnosing the Deepest Level of Imbalance

Ji Zu De Na Gu Ka. Like a mantra, this is the string of sound images we will repeat again and again, patient after patient, at the beginning of a treatment, at the end, and somewhere in between, in order to determine which meridian system is currently engaged in the task of maintaining or restoring this patient's health.

As you will find in your *Reference Manual*, "Ji" is the sound image associated with the Regular Meridian system. "Zu" is the sound image for the Extra Meridian system; "De" is for the Divergent, "Na" is for the Oceans System; "Gu" and "Ka" are associated with the two levels of the Cosmic Meridians system.

It is good to practice this now, even if you have not yet learned the treatment protocols for each system.

> **Instruction**
> Diagnosing the deepest level of imbalance
>
> 1. With your patient lying face up, place your palm over their tanden, and while performing the finger test, image the sounds associated with each meridian system: "Ji, Zu, De, Na, Gu, Ka." You can also check these levels from the patient's back, placing your sensor hand at the upper lumbar level.
>
> 2. The sound images will elicit a sticky response for energy systems that are out of balance. For example, if your finger test reads sticky when you image the sound "Ji" and smooth for the remaining sound images, you will need to address only the Regular Meridian system. If the finger test reads sticky at "Zu," but smooth for the sound image "De," you will know that the deepest imbalance is being manifested in the Extra Meridians. And so on. If the finger test elicits a sticky response for the sound image "De," but smooth at "Na," then you know that the deepest imbalance lies in the Divergent Meridians.

Determining a Focus:
Structural or Internal

Knowing whether the patient's issues are primarily structural ones or internal ones – emotional/organic – helps us decide which treatment goals to focus on and which treatment method to use.

> **Instruction**
> Determining a structural or internal treatment focus
>
> 1. After you have cleared surface ja ki from your patient and immediately after you have diagnosed your patient's deepest level of imbalance, place your general sensor on the inside (palm) of your patient's open hand. Finger test while imaging the question: is the patient's problem primarily internal? If the response is sticky, the answer is yes; if the response is smooth, the answer is no.
>
> 2. Double check by finger testing the back of the patient's hand and imaging the question: is the patient's problem mainly structural? Sticky means yes, smooth means no.

Locating Specific Structural Problems

Misaligned joints, muscle strains, inflamed ligaments, bruises — anything that affects the "hardware" of the body whether or not it is visible to the naked eye, palpable with the hand, or something we are able to name in medical terms — can be clearly detected via the body's meridian system and the language of energy. While structural problems can sometimes be remedied with a honji treatment, they usually need the specific attention that a hyoji treatment gives. In Chapter 6, you will learn how the Extra Meridians play a major role in the structural alignment of the human body. The simple diagnostic method outlined below, which combines sound imaging and the finger test, will help you to locate very specific structural imbalances. Eventually, you will learn to identify their patterns, and select from a variety of treatment approaches.

> **Instruction**
> Locating specific structural problems
>
> 1. To find your patient's main structural problem or problems, scan their body with an open palm, image the sound "Ne," and finger test. A sticky sensation gives you the general location of a structural problem. The chances are good you will locate more than one such area producing a sticky result.
>
> 2. Once you have located the general area of the problem, you may wish to use a pointed tool such as a chopstick to further localize it.

Shin So Shiatsu and Diode Treatment

In my training as an electrical engineer I never imagined that diodes — components in radios, televisions, and computers — would be useful in treatment of the human body. Diodes are tiny semiconductors (some 6 millimetres or 2.5 inches long) whose function is to move electrical current in a given direction and rectify power supply. Therapy using diodes was developed about a quarter of a century ago by the Japanese acupuncturist Dr. Yoshio Manaka and his research group.

My years of research and treatment with diodes have taught me that they are effective and simple to use. They are inexpensive, and create no side effects. I use them in conjunction with Shin So Shiatsu especially for alleviating muscle and joint pain, and in living spaces, to seal off areas where ja ki emanates from the ground (see below).

I work with both silicone and germanium diodes. In the therapeutic context, I have found the silicon diodes work faster, while the benefits of germanium diodes are longer lasting. These are available through some retailers of electronic equipment, and in bulk, through wholesalers. I recommend diodes numbered IN60 or a similar capacity.

To avoid injury or discomfort to the patient, curl the ends of your diode as shown in figure 4-2.

Ja ki often presents itself in our work and living spaces. Using the finger test, we can easily detect where it rises from beneath the surface of the floor. This ja ki can disrupt our sleep, our general sense of well-being, and our Shin So diagnoses.

Treatment Responses

Shin So Shiatsu provides us with very powerful tools for improving a patient's condition. It is important to keep in mind that clearing internal ja ki and treating meridian systems at the deeper levels may produce notable treatment responses — or *men ken* — in the first hours or days after the treatment. These reactions, which are variable, often include a temporary return or exacerbation of symptoms. This can be considered a positive result, but it is wise nonetheless to prepare the patient for this possible aspect of their healing journey.

In the meantime, as therapists we must also develop a clear sense of when a treatment is complete. And as we progress with the various stages of a treatment, we must pay careful attention not to over stimulate the patient.

Instruction
Using diodes with Shin So Shiatsu

1. Locate the structural problem or painful area(s). See steps 1-2, "locating structural problems," above.

2. Place a diode directly on the stickiest spot(s), and parallel with vertical meridian flow in that particular area. Finger test again while rotating the diode in four directions: three of these positions will elicit a sticky response; only one, the most effective location for the diode, will read smooth.

3. Tape the diode in place and finger test again to ensure a smooth reading.

4. Finger test areas above and below the diode: often two and sometimes more diodes are needed to address a particular structural problem.

Note: If you are working with a diode and find that it elicits a sticky response in all four directions, the diode may be defective. Try another one.

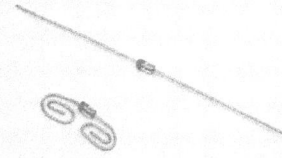

Figure 4-2 A diode. To avoid injury or discomfort to the patient, curl the ends of your diode as shown here.

Instruction
Sealing off a ja ki source in a room

1. Tape a diode to a small piece of cardboard.

2. Place a strong substance such as a few cigarettes or painkillers in one hand: finger test to confirm a very sticky negative response. Now, with substances in hand, move slowly around the room and continue finger testing. When you encounter the negative energy of a ja ki source, the finger test will suddenly shift from being sticky to smooth.

3. Place the diode on the floor here, and rotate it 360 degrees while performing the finger test. Tape the cardboard and diode into position when you get a sticky response.

4. Finger test and place a diode under your treatment mat (beneath the receiver's low back area) and another one beneath the spot where you perform most of your diagnostic work.

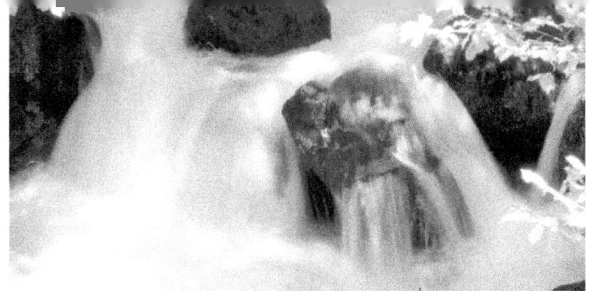

5

Diagnosing and Treating
The Regular Meridians

blown to the big river
floating away
cherry blossoms

- Issa Kobayashi -

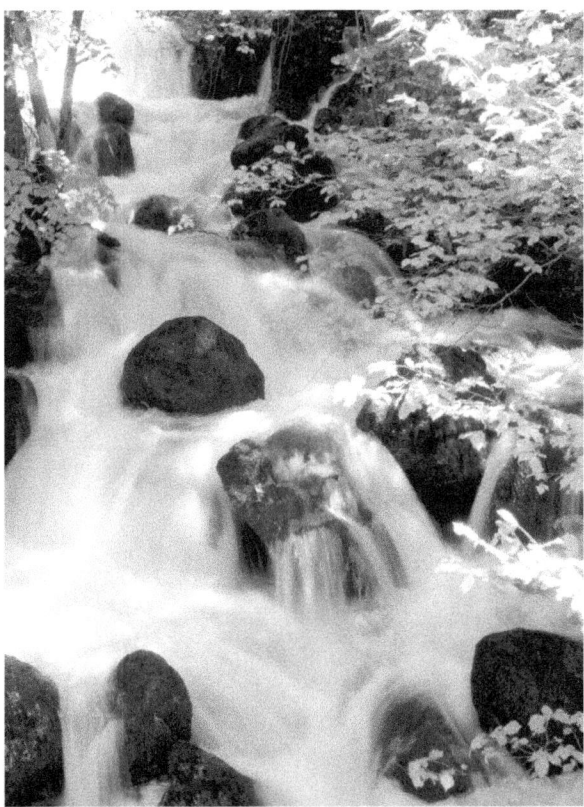

In this chapter, you will learn:

- How to diagnose Regular Meridian imbalances.

- How to confirm your diagnoses.

- How to treat Regular Meridian imbalances using shiatsu.

- How to treat Shin So Master Points.

Chapter 5

Diagnosing and Treating
The Regular Meridians

Shiatsu therapists and practitioners of other meridian-based therapies have tended to focus only on the Regular Meridian system, sometimes referred to as the "main" meridians. In Shin So Shiatsu, whether or not imbalances are identified in the deeper meridian systems, thorough diagnosis and treatment of the Regular Meridian system is essential.

In approaching the Regular Meridians, we are mainly concerned with identifying which pathways have reached a third-degree imbalance, and of these, which one is the most kyo and which one is the most jitsu. For a more complete picture of the patient's condition, we also pay attention, particularly, to second-degree imbalances. At this point, you may wish to review Chapter 1 for an in-depth description of the Regular Meridians at all three levels.

Regular Meridians in First Degree

First-degree meridians are already in a state of balance. All 12 Regular Meridians will ideally fall into this category after a treatment. When this degree of balance can be sustained, the body is more able to heal itself.

Regular Meridians in Second Degree

Second-degree imbalances tend to reflect our patients' complaints — their awareness and expression of physical or emotional discomfort. For example, if our patient reports headaches or eye-related issues, irritation or frustration, we may find that the Liver Meridian is manifesting a second-degree jitsu imbalance. It may be that the Kidney Meridian is most kyo in third degree, and therefore unable to support the Liver energy. In other words, while kyo and jitsu meridians at third degree are not always clearly linked to the patient's complaints, treating them is vital for rebalancing and rejuvenating the Regular Meridian system at its deepest point of imbalance. Figure 5-1 illustrates this.

It is important to remember, however, that there will be times when the patient's complaint is not reflected in our diagnosis of their most kyo-jitsu meridian in second-degree. The meridian system itself may be "reporting" hidden symptoms — something the patient may not even be aware of.

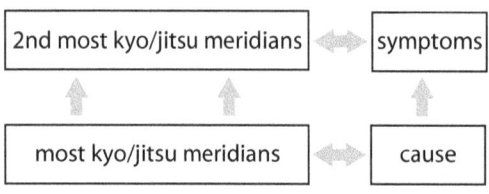

Figure 5-1 Relationship between meridian imbalance and symptoms

Regular Meridians in Third Degree

Diagnosing the most kyo and jitsu meridians at the third-degree level gives us the information we need to treat and balance the entire Regular Meridian system.

Balancing meridian energy (sei ki) does not necessarily mean the patient's symptoms will disappear. For example, in cancer patients, the meridian systems may be balanced after a good treatment, but the cancer is still present. Balanced energy indicates the patient's system is working with maximum efficiency to eliminate a problem. But when the force of an illness is very strong, the ki-meridian system can easily be knocked out of balance. It is important that our treatments occur at sufficient intervals to maximize how long the patient is in a balanced energetic state.

The Regular Meridians are very dynamic and can shift from one level of imbalance to another over a period of even a few hours, especially in those suffering serious illnesses. This is why it is so important we fine tune our ability to communicate with the body's energy systems. With the finger test, we become very sensitive to changes in our patients' energy states. We see how quickly their meridian systems revert to deeper levels of imbalance after a treatment. And then, we can recommend appropriate intervals for treatments.

Four Key Meridians

TCM associates each of the three sources of ki with a particular meridian function.

Types of (Sei) Ki	Associated Meridian
Prenatal ki	Kidney (Bladder)
Ki from food and drinks	Stomach (Spleen)
Ki from the air	Large Intestine (Lung)

When we hear of the ki we receive from air, we may logically assume this means oxygen. However, it is more accurate to say that air in this case refers to the broader concept of Cosmic energy. Cosmic energy is absorbed through our skin: a function carried out largely by the Large Intestine Meridian.

While each of the 12 Regular Meridians plays a critical role in helping us maintain a balanced state of health, the Kidney, Stomach, and Large Intestine meridians are most essential to life in their production and integration of ki from the three sources described above. But practically speaking, one more meridian must be added to this trio. It is not enough just to have ki. Ki must also be distributed to where it is needed. This is the Liver Meridian's job.

When these four meridians are functioning optimally, we enjoy a basic level of health, i.e. at the first-degree level.

It is important to note that, ideally, the Stomach and Kidney meridians will reflect a more kyo energy state, while the Large Intestine and the Liver meridians will ideally be more jitsu. When this is so, and all four of these meridians are in the first-degree state, you will not find any imbalance in the other eight meridians.

Diagnosing the Regular Meridians:
Kyo and Jitsu

A key piece of information in diagnosing the Regular Meridians is which are the most kyo and which are the most jitsu in nature. As students of Zen Shiatsu, we learned to use gentle hand or finger pressure on the hara diagnostic zones to determine this. However, because this part of the body reflects so many degrees or levels of information, reliable results are usually difficult to obtain. Adding to the confusion are the intestines, manifesting various degrees of hardness or softness not directly related to energy quality, and affecting palpation of any part of the abdomen.

Instruction
Diagnosing kyo and jitsu

1. Identify the diagnostic zone you wish to find. For example, if you wish to find the Stomach Meridian diagnostic zone, use your general sensor to locate it on either the patient's back or hara.

2. Hold your sensor finger — in this case, the index finger of your right hand — about three inches above the patient's body, and point it toward the Stomach Meridian diagnostic zone (see figure 5-2).

3. Maintain a clear image: you are diagnosing the Stomach Meridian, and you want to know whether this meridian's energy is kyo or jitsu in quality.

4. If the finger test feels smooth, the Stomach Meridian is kyo; if it feels sticky, it is jitsu.

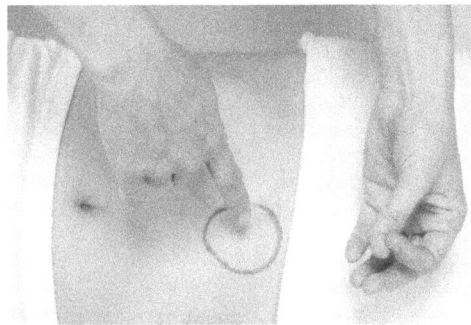

Figure 5-2 Diagnosing kyo and jitsu

Confirming our Shin So Diagnosis

A major advantage of the Shin So Shiatsu approach is that we are able to diagnose a particular meridian or meridian system as being out of balance, and then immediately confirm that diagnosis. In this case, you have just diagnosed a meridian as being the most kyo or most jitsu in the third degree. Now, you can confirm that result. As you begin, it is important to remember to keep your mind as clear as possible: clinging to your initial diagnosis, or conversely, clouding your mind with doubt about your diagnosis, will undermine the confirmation method.

Instruction
Confirming a kyo-jitsu diagnosis

1. Hold a small piece of aluminum foil about three inches above the diagnostic zone and finger test (see figure 5-3). Smooth is kyo; sticky is jitsu.

2. Now, palpate the hara zone with your hands. This helps develop confidence and sensitize your fingers to these kyo and jitsu qualities of energy.

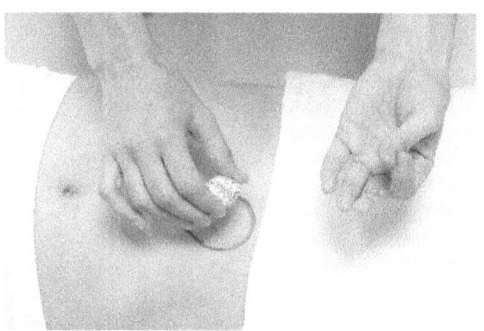

Figure 5-3 Using aluminum foil to confirm our kyo-jitsu diagnosis.

Instruction
Diagnosing which third-degree meridians need treatment

1. With your patient lying comfortably face down or face up, place your third-degree sensor about two inches above the diagnostic area (see figure 5-4). Refer to your Saito back diagnostic chart or abdominal chart of first-degree diagnostic zones (figures 2-2a, 2-8g, and *Reference Manual*).

2. Performing the finger test, slowly scan each of the 12 diagnostic zones with your third-degree sensor. At the same time, be sure to image the meridian name corresponding to each diagnostic zone. Two zones will feel distinctly sticky. These correlate to the meridians "active" in third-degree imbalance.

3. Diagnose each of these two zone's energy quality (see "diagnosing a Regular Meridian as kyo or jitsu," above).

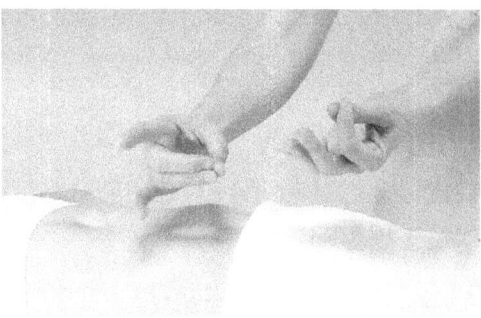

Figure 5-4 Finger testing the abdomen: we can use the third-degree sensor and the first-degree diagnostic zone.

Instruction
Diagnosing the most imbalanced second-degree meridians

1. Follow the steps outlined above for diagnosing a third-degree imbalance, but this time use your second-degree sensor (figure 5-5). This diagnosis will reinforce information you have about the patient's complaints.

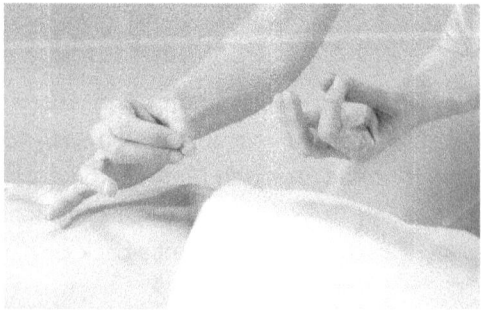

Figure 5-5 This sensor is used to diagnose meridians in second-degree imbalance.

Instruction
Confirming your diagnosis of a third-degree yin meridian

When any of the six yin meridians reach the third-degree of imbalance, its flow shifts to the back of the body. This is easily detected with the finger test. To confirm your yin meridian diagnosis, you check the energy flow at the patient's sacrum (see figure 5-6). For example, if you have determined that the Kidney Meridian is manifesting a third-degree imbalance, either kyo or jitsu:

1. Position your general sensor one to two inches above the patient's Governing Vessel at the sacrum.

2. Move your sensor hand slowly toward the lateral edge of the sacrum while performing the finger test.

3. Image the meridian name (Kidney Meridian).

4. If your initial diagnosis was correct, your tester will feel sticky as it picks up the Kidney Meridian's third-degree flow near the edge of the sacrum. If your tester feels smooth, your initial diagnosis was incorrect.

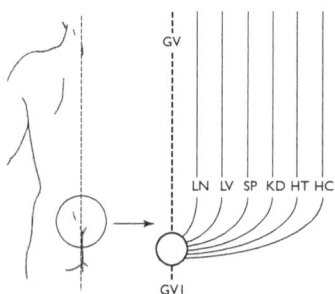

Figure 5-6 To confirm our diagnosis of yin Regular Meridians in third degree we check the sacrum area.

Instruction
Confirming your diagnosis of a third-degree yang meridian

To confirm a third-degree diagnosis of any of the six yang meridians we follow the procedure described above for the yin meridians, but check the energy flow at the back of the patient's neck, as shown in figure 5-7.

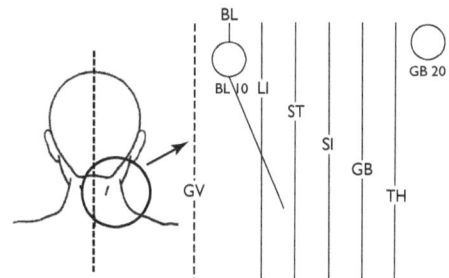

Figure 5-7 To confirm our diagnosis of yang Regular Meridians in third degree we check the meridians at the back of the neck.

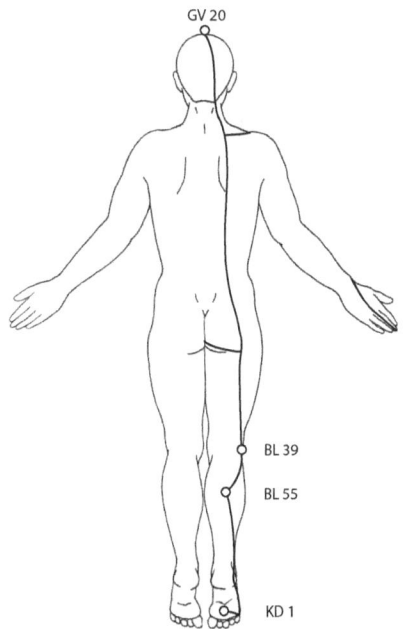

Figure 5-8 You can also confirm a diagnosis of the Bladder Meridian in third-degree by checking for energy flowing laterally along the back.

Treating the Regular Meridians

Some patients will manifest imbalances in only the Regular Meridian system, while their deeper meridian systems remain unaffected. These individuals are usually in good health, mentally and physically, or are effectively dealing with a condition through diet, exercise, or some other form of therapy. In these instances, our treatment need only focus on the Regular Meridian system.

The two main components in Shin So Shiatsu's approach to the Regular Meridians are the honji treatment, followed by the hyoji treatment (see Chapter 4).

Honji Treatment

As I said in Chapter 4, we can compare our purpose here to building a good house foundation. We focus on the patient's deepest level of imbalance. In the context of a Regular Meridian treatment, this means treating and balancing the most kyo meridian and the most jitsu meridian. To accomplish this, Shin So Shiatsu applies the basic techniques of Zen Shiatsu. Our goal is to achieve a state of meridian balance that lasts as long as possible in order to maximize the body's chances to heal itself.

Hyoji Treatment

The hyoji treatment addresses what we identify as the patient's main symptom or problem area. Shin So Shiatsu methods include shiatsu pressure, the yaki hari technique, and the use of diodes and acupuncture press needles.

Magnetic Polarity of the Sensor

Our bodies are microcosms of the universe around us, and in keeping with this, is the observation that the energy flow in each of our fingers corresponds to a magnetic polarity. In most people, the right index finger possesses north-pole energy and the left index finger possesses south-pole energy.

The north pole functions to tonify energy; the south pole sedates energy. The energy of abdominal diagnostic zones (and all energy circles) can be characterized as either kyo or jitsu in nature. Let's say, for example, the Heart Meridian diagnostic zone is kyo. This means it needs tonification. When you place your north-pole finger near this zone, it accepts the tonifying energy, so that when we finger test, we get a smooth response. If we were to place our middle, or south-pole finger near this kyo zone, it would reject the sedative energy. With the finger test, we would get a sticky response.

A few individuals demonstrate "reversed" polarities (i.e. the right index finger possesses south-pole energy, and the left possesses north-pole energy) and the finger test must be interpreted accordingly.

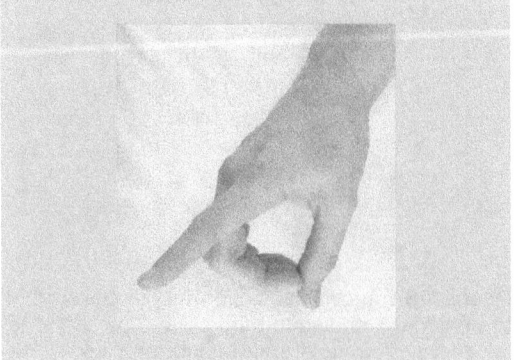

Belt Zones and Stretch Positions

In Chapter 2, I described how my discovery of the meridian belt zones resolved questions about how Masunaga's meridian stretch positions were linked to the treatment of meridians.

To recap: figure 5-9a shows the location of the Regular Meridian belt zones; we can see the Liver Meridian located at the top of the thigh, close to the level of the hip joints. Figure 5-9b shows the stretch positions for the Liver Meridian in second and third degree. When you place the patient's heel at the lower border of the Liver Meridian belt zone, the Liver Meridian begins to flow in the pattern of a second-degree imbalance. When you place the patient's heel at the upper border of the belt zone and test for the meridian location, third-degree flow appears.

In a Shin So Shiatsu treatment, one first diagnoses the degree of energy imbalance in the meridians, then positions the leg according to that diagnosis. Accuracy in placing the heel against either border of the meridian belt zone is paramount. A centimetre of error can significantly affect the treatment outcome. Therefore, it is important to confirm the location of the meridian flow once the patient is positioned for treatment.

It is also helpful to note that these stretch positions influence the body's energy in the hip joint and pelvic area, rather than the knee joint. Once you have ensured the leg opens from the hip in the correct position, the knee can be straightened and the lower leg opened outwards to enhance both the patient's comfort and your access to the meridians.

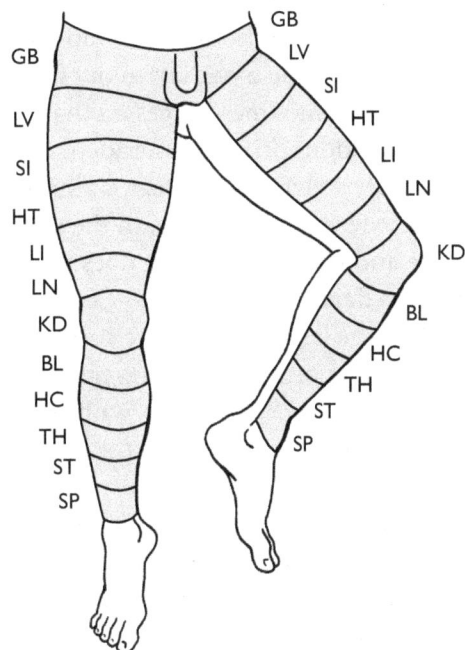

Figure 5-9a Regular Meridian belt zones

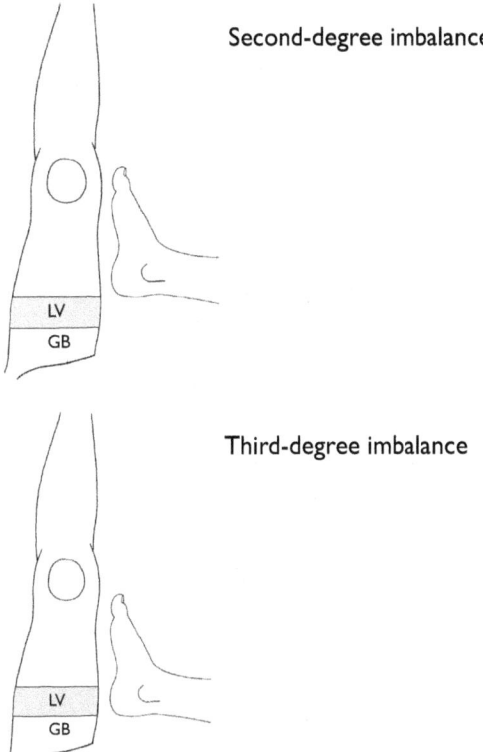

Figure 5-9b Stretch position for the Liver Meridian

Another advantage of these stretch positions is that they reveal more clearly the kyo or jitsu condition of the muscle through which the meridian in question travels. It is sometimes suggested that the stretch positions bring the meridian closer to the body's surface. The Regular Meridians, however, run just beneath the skin's surface and stretching the leg does not affect the depth of ki flow.

When the legs and arms are correctly positioned, another fascinating phenomenon takes place. We are able, with the finger test, to detect two ja ki points (Shin So Ja Ki Points) on each leg and arm — points which have "opened up" in order to recieve fresh ki, and which in turn will facilitate the release of ja ki from the meridian channel. These ja ki holes are similar in nature to the two holes we find on the front of the body when we are undertaking to clear surface ja ki (Chapter 3). Here, in working with the meridians, should you shift the limb position even slightly, these ja ki points will close up again.

Instruction
Positioning the arm for Regular Meridian treatment

1. With your hand in the third-degree sensor position, firmly grasp the patient's arm near the wrist and fully extend the arm above the shoulder.

2. Gently slide it downward while imaging the name of the meridian you need to find.

3. When the arm is correctly positioned, the finger test will feel sticky. Use the chart in figure 5-11 to help guide you.

Instruction
Positioning the leg for Regular Meridian treatment

The order in which the meridian belt zones appear on the leg corresponds exactly to Masunaga's meridian stretch positions. Memorizing the chart of meridian belt zones facilitates quick positioning for treatment: this should be followed by confirmation with the finger test.

1. With your hand in the third-degree sensor position, firmly grasp the patient's leg near the ankle (figure 5-10).

2. Gently slide the leg upward as far as possible (it's easier to start from the top) and then downward, while imaging the name of the meridian you are looking for.

When the leg is correctly positioned, the finger test will feel sticky.

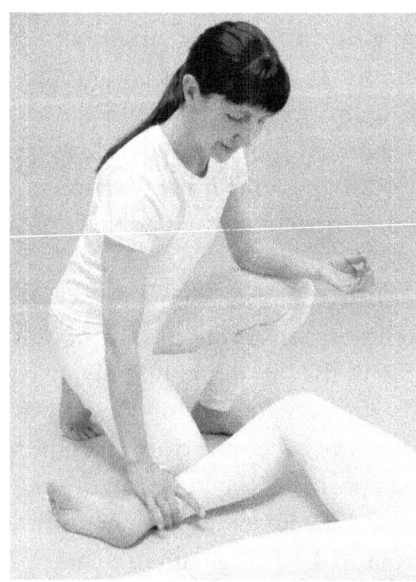

Figure 5-10 Positioning the leg to treat the meridians in third degree.

Instruction
Confirming correct leg and arm positioning

Our example here is the Heart Meridian in third degree with treatment first focussed on the leg.

1. Make sure that the third-degree sensor feels sticky over the Heart Meridian diagnostic zone (refer to the first-degree abdominal diagnostic chart).

2. Position the leg for treatment of the Heart Meridian in third degree.

3. Return to the diagnostic zone and repeat the finger test.

4. If the patient's leg is correctly positioned, finger testing with the third-degree sensor will elicit a smooth sensation; finger testing with the first-degree sensor elicits a sticky response.

Once you have treated the Heart Meridian on the legs, and are about to treat the same meridian on the arm, it is important to consider the following:

1. Having treated the Heart Meridian on the legs, the Heart Meridian will become balanced (first degree). Finger testing the Heart Meridian diagnostic zone with your third-degree sensor will elicit a smooth response; with the first-degree sensor, you will get a sticky response.

2. However, to stabilize the meridian's balanced condition, you must follow through by treating the Heart Meridian on the arm. First, you position the arm according to the chart (figure 5-11); then, to confirm the position is correct, finger test with your third-degree sensor. You should get a sticky response.

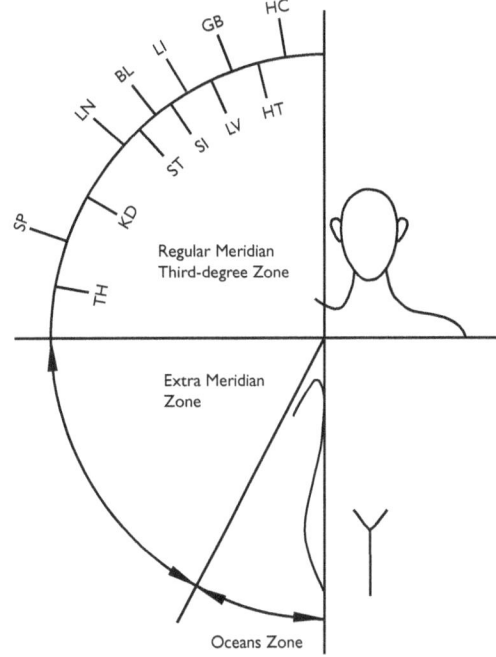

Figure 5-11 Arm positions for 12 Regular Meridians in third-degree imbalance. Regular Meridian positions are above the shoulder, toward the head.

The Importance of Treating Meridians on the Arms and Legs

Which part of the body is more important to treat? No book can tell us. This depends on the patient: we must sense and concentrate on areas where the energy flow is interrupted. Generally speaking however, the back, abdominal areas, legs, and arms require a lot of attention.

My exploration of the meridian belt zones confirmed for me how important the arms and legs are, and how they represent the energy of the whole body (see figure 2-13). We can see how the appearance of the meridian zones corresponds to the locations of the anatomical organs (this is especially true of the Divergent Meridian belt zones, and as we will learn in Chapter 7, the Divergent Meridians link directly to the organs). This may explain why, on the TCM chart, so many important acupuncture points are located along the arms and legs. Shin So Shiatsu treatments also concentrate on these energetically intense areas. This is reflected in figure 2-12, with the third-degree Regular Meridians on the arm and leg.

Instruction
Treating the most kyo and jitsu meridians on the arm and leg

As much has been taught and written on this subject, here I will only briefly outline treatment positions recommended for Shin So Shiatsu. Specific positions for each meridian are illustrated in your *Reference Manual*.

Yin/yang Regular Meridian treatment on the arm

With the patient supine, we can easily position the arm for treatment of the six yin meridians. The six yang meridians are easily accessed with the patient lying prone, or face down, and arms outstretched.

Yin/yang Regular Meridian treatment on the leg

With the patient supine we can position the leg to treat five yin meridians (all but the Lung Meridian) as well as the Small Intestine meridian. We fix their particular position as shown in figure 5-10, ensuring that when treating the leg, the knee is open as much as possible. The Lung Meridian in third-degree is treated with patient in side position. The five yang meridians (all but the Small Intestine Meridian) can be treated very comfortably with the patient in side position.

Shin So Shiatsu Master Points

Shin So Shiatsu Master Points are quick and effective tools for reducing muscular tension along a meridian path. There are three major sets of Master Points.

1. **At the back of the axilla, near the acupuncture point SI 9.**
   Gently supporting this point at the back of the upper arm, while treating the neck and shoulder area (see figure 5-12), will help reduce muscular tension.

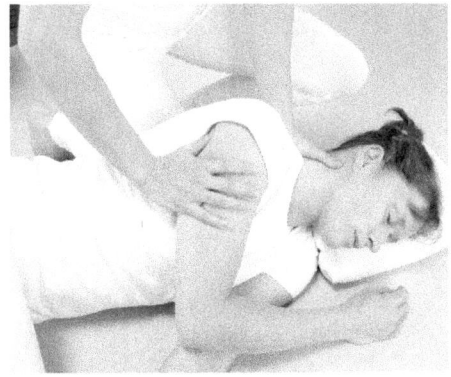

Figure 5-12 Neck and shoulder treatment

2. **Bladder points on the sacrum.**
   Treating Bladder Meridian points along the sacrum helps reduce back tension. We start by treating points along the patient's back, working both sides simultaneously, from top to bottom, at least once. Then we gently position our middle fingers on Bladder Meridian points 27 and 28, holding each point on both sides simultaneously for two to three minutes. Returning to the back treatment, we will notice how much more easily any residual tension releases (see figure 5-13).

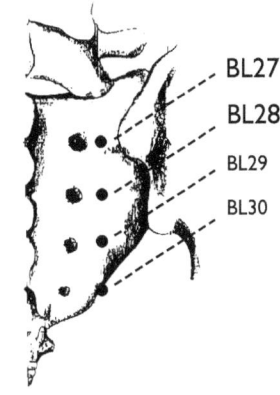

Figure 5-13 Master Points on the sacrum

3. **At the back of legs, just below the hips.**
   These points (figure 5-14) help remove tension in the lower legs. The therapist can use either the thumbs or elbow, while letting the other hand rest gently on the same leg.

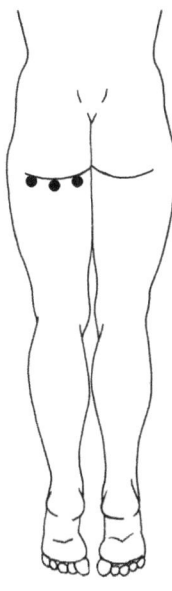

Figure 5-14 Master Points on the back of the legs

6

Diagnosing and Treating
The Extra Meridians

spring day…
a long line of footprints
on the sandy beach

- Shiki Masaoka -

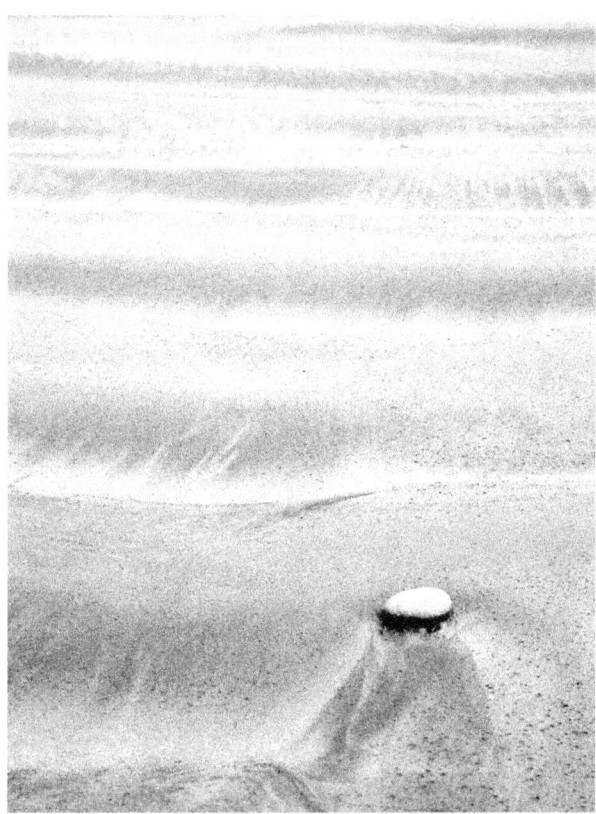

In this chapter, you will learn:

- How the Extra Meridians relate to the Regular Meridians.

- How to sense Extra Meridians, their belt zones and energy circles.

- How to diagnose imbalances in the Extra Meridian system.

- How to find Extra Meridian Confluent Points and use them in treatment.

- How to treat Extra Meridians using yaki hari, shiatsu, ja ki removal, and ion pumping methods.

- How to diagnose and treat structural problems associated with Extra Meridian imbalances.

- How to locate acupuncture points.

Chapter 6

Diagnosing and Treating
The Extra Meridians

When we hear of Extra Meridians, we might think they are something extra, or extraneous to the Regular Meridians. There's so little mention of them after all. How important can they be?

Or we might infer from their name that these pathways are actually very important — because they pick up the extra or over flow from the Regular or "main stream" of ki and carry it to the "ocean." And this is in fact their primary and vital function, as we shall explore in this chapter.

The Chinese name for these Extra Meridians — *ki kei* — suggests there is even more to know of this system's remarkable functions and behaviours. *Kei* means meridian, and *ki*, here, denotes something "strange," "abnormal," "unusual," or "mysterious." As my exploration of the Extra Meridians progressed, I began to appreciate why they have been characterized as such. I have come to think of them as the Extraordinary Meridians, which they are also sometimes called.

When the Regular Meridians cannot regulate the body's energy on their own, these extraordinary Extra Meridians become involved. The minor Extra Meridian imbalances we experience in our daily lives can often be regulated through a Regular Meridian treatment protocol. But in cases of more serious imbalances — whether acute or chronic and whether experienced on a physical or emotional level — a Regular Meridian treatment will not be enough. To ensure a positive response and to prevent recurrence of the problem, we must treat the Extra Meridian system directly. Treatments combining both the Regular and Extra Meridian systems yield the most powerful results.

As with Regular Meridians, much of my research into this system has involved salvaging lost knowledge: existing fragments strongly suggest that a much more comprehensive body of information once existed. Over the past two decades, there has been renewed interest in the Extra Meridians, particularly in Japan, with most emphasis being placed on treatment via the hatsu-so-ketsu or Confluent Points. But the development of practical applications for this energy system lags far behind that of the Regular Meridians. I believe the main reason for this has been the absence of detailed charts for all but the Governor and Conception vessels. We have been working in the dark: our understanding of when, where, why, and how energy transfers between systems, or even which Regular Meridians flow into which Extra Meridians, has been limited.

Thus my first goal as I embarked on this next phase of my research was to locate and chart the Extra Meridians as completely as possible using the Finger Test Method. It was obvious from the outset that my newly supplemented knowledge of the Regular Meridians was essential for exploring the connections between these two systems.

In the process, I discovered Extra Meridian belt zones and energy circles (see Chapter 2), both of which will be discussed in detail. Subsequently, I focussed on developing diagnostic techniques and practical applications especially suitable for shiatsu professionals and others working with the ki-meridian systems.

The TCM View

Following is a summary of what TCM tells us about Extra Meridian functions, locations, and access points.

- There are eight Extra Meridians, as shown in figure 6-1.

Yang Meridians	Yin Meridians
Governor Vessel Du Mai	Conception Vessel Ren Mai
Yang Connecting Meridian Yang Wei Mai	Yin Connecting Meridian Yin Wei Mai
Belt Meridian Dai Mai	Penetrating Meridian Chong Mai
Yang Heel Meridian Yang Qiao Mai	Yin Heel Meridian Yin Qiao Mai

Figure 6-1 The Extra Meridians

- While the Regular Meridians connect directly to the internal organs, the Extra Meridians do not.

- The Extra Meridians' main function is to receive ki overflow from the Regular Meridians. The Extra Meridians are often likened to a reservoir that draws excess water from ditches and canals in times of heavy rain. This is how they help regulate the Regular Meridian system.

- Except for the Conception and Governor vessel, Extra Meridians do not have their own acupuncture points. However, the Extra Meridians have long been treated in acupuncture through the use of Confluent Points. Each meridian has its Confluent Point, and this point is treated in conjunction with another. Figure 6-2 describes this pairing for treatment purposes.

Extra Meridians	Treatment Points
Governor Vessel Yang Heel Meridian	SI 3 BL 62
Belt Meridian Yang Connecting Meridian	GB 41 TH 5
Conception Vessel Yin Heel Meridian	LU 7 KD 6
Penetrating Meridian Yin Connecting Meridian	SP 4 HC 6

Figure 6-2 Extra Meridian Confluent Points

Toward a More Complete Picture

In tracing the pathways of the eight Extra Meridians, I found my results largely agreed with those of Japanese acupuncturists Tsutomu Kishi, Y. Nagahama M.D., and A. Maruyama, M.D. More research will no doubt begin to resolve the discrepancies that do exist.

In the process of my work, foremost in my mind was at what point do imbalances in the Regular Meridians activate the Extra Meridian system. My clinical research

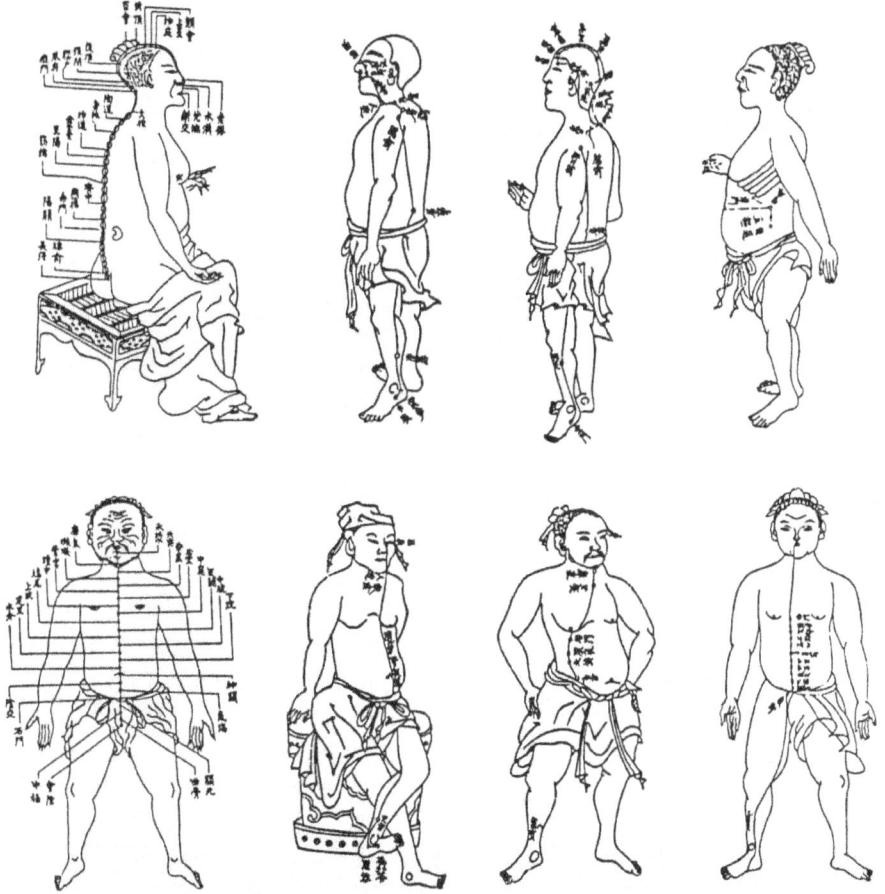

Figure 6-3 TCM charts such as this illustrate the Extra Meridians. While both the Conception and Governor channels are clearly shown, it seems to me that the mapping of the six remaining Extra Meridians has remained incomplete.

revealed that this transfer of energy occurs when a Regular Meridian has reached the third degree, or sho-sei-byo level of imbalance. Or, more precisely, once a Regular Meridian has reached a third-degree imbalance, and the imbalance is still increasing to the point that the Regular Meridian system can no longer contain it, then the jitsu quality of energy is siphoned off and flows into the Extra Meridian system; the kyo quality of energy eventually flows into the Divergent Meridian system, as illustrated in figure 6-4. Furthermore, once this transfer takes place, the Regular Meridian that overflows into the Extra Meridians drops to a second-level or ze-do-byo imbalance.

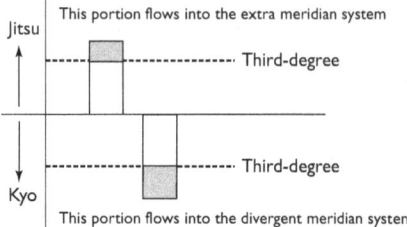

Figure 6-4

A Note on Extra Meridian Names

While in Shin So Shiatsu we emphasize sensing rather than memorizing the meridian pathways, a basic understanding of their functions and routes is vital to developing a working relationship with them. Meridian-based shiatsu therapists, most familiar with the Regular Meridians, are already able to associate the names of these vessels with their functions and their routes, always an important aid in remembering them.

A scarcity of material in English and limited experience with the deeper meridian systems makes understanding and working with them more difficult. Fortunately, the Divergent Meridians share the same function-related names as their Regular Meridian counterparts. For a richer explanation of Extra Meridians names and functions, I recommend *Extraordinary Vessels* (Kiiko Matsumoto, and Stephen Birch, Paradigm Publications, Brooklyn, 1986). The following brief explanation of Extra Meridian names (in English followed by their TCM names) is designed to help you remember them.

- **Governor Vessel (Du Mai):** The Governor and Conception vessels are traditionally said to govern the Regular Meridians.
- **Conception Vessel (Ren Mai):** In addition to its governing role, this vessel is associated in proximity and function to the reproductive system and pregnancy.
- **Penetrating Meridian (Chong Mai):** Where one form of energy meets another and creates something new, implying the action of penetration (sexual intercourse) leading to pregnancy. The Penetrating Meridian is said to connect pre- and post-natal ki. The classics also mention its role in the production of Defensive Ki. My own research has found that the Triple Heater Regular Meridian, which is associated with the sexual organs and Defensive Ki, overflows into the Penetrating Extra Meridian.
- **Belt Meridian (Dai Mai):** This meridian, which encircles the abdomen like a belt, regulates the Extra Meridians.
- **Yin and Yang Heel Meridians (Yin Qiao Mai, Yang Qiao Mai):** Flow to the heel or ankle area, and influence the movement of the limbs.
- **Yin and Yang Connecting Meridians (Yang Wei Mai, Yin Wei Mai):** These structurally unusual meridians (figures 6-9 and 6-10, below) connect the six yin and yang Regular Meridians and carry their overflow.

Hatsu-so-ketsu:
Confluent Points

TCM identifies special hatsu-so-ketsu or Confluent Points which help us access and regulate the Extra Meridians. A quick study of today's TCM charts offers no clues as to why these points were originally selected, although their effectiveness has been proven again and again in clinical use. While it is likely that more complete charts of the Extra Meridians once existed, it is also likely that practitioners of days gone by were exceptionally sensitive to this ki-energy system and were simply able to "feel" these highly effective points in their day-to-day work.

In charting the Extra Meridians, their relationships to each other and their links via Confluent Points become clear. We can see how close certain Extra Meridians are to each other — they lie almost side by side. We can see that these particular meridians intersect, and it is at these intersections that Confluent Points are situated. For example, the Yang Heel and Governing meridians cross each other at Confluent Points SI 3 and BL 62. All of the Confluent Points for the Extra Meridians are located below the elbows and knees where the ki flow is most dynamic. When the Extra Meridian system is activated by an excess of energy from the Regular Meridian system, these points can be used to discharge or redistribute the excess energy.

Where They Flow:
The Extra Meridians

According to my research, once the Regular Meridian system has reached the third level of imbalance, the Extra Meridians engage in the remarkable flow pattern that gives them the name *ki kei*. To begin with, all yin Regular Meridians overflow into yang Extra Meridians. All yang Regular Meridians overflow into yin Extra Meridians. This has great implications in terms of understanding the direction of energy flow within the Extra Meridian system: that is to say, it is totally reversed from that of the Regular Meridians. Keeping in mind that yin Regular Meridians flow upward in the body, and that the function of the Extra Meridians is to handle the excess flow of energy from this system, it then follows that the energy flow within the yang Extra Meridians would also be upward. Similarly, within the yin Extra Meridian system, the flow will be downward, as these meridians receive excess ki from the yang Regular Meridians. Figure 6-5 illustrates this.

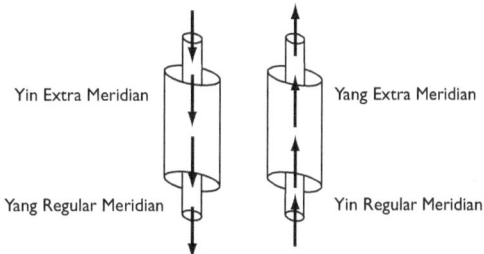

Figure 6-5

Furthermore, this excess energy from the yin Regular Meridians flows to the yang aspect of the body, while the yang Regular Meridians overflow to the yin aspect of the body. This points to another remarkable feature of the Extra Meridians as they relate to the Regular Meridians: their role in helping preserve the body's structural integrity. For example, figure 6-6 shows how the excessive flow of energy in the Spleen Meridian activates the Yang Connecting Meridian.

We can see how these two meridians run symmetrically up the yin and yang sides of the body. I believe this rerouting

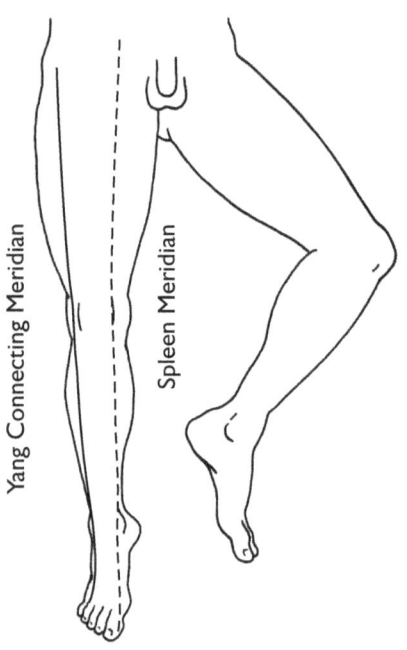

Figure 6-6 The excess flow of energy in the Spleen Meridian activates the Yang Connecting Meridian.

of excess energy assists us in maintaining functional structural integrity under less than ideal circumstances. Should the energy overflow traverse the same side of the body as the imbalanced Regular Meridian, the ensuing muscle tension and other structural changes could become a source of distress. This is just one more example of how absolutely complex and fascinating the meridian systems are in regulating our overall energetic make-up.

Links between the Regular and Extra Meridians

My research to date supports the meridian-to-meridian relationships specified below in figure 6-7.

The Connecting Meridians

The Yang Connecting and Yin Connecting Extra Meridians (figure 6-8) form a wide band of energy flowing along the leg.

One of the most interesting features of this particular widening of the Extra Meridians is that, with the finger test, we can feel the energies of each of the six Regular Meridians flowing within these bands. This energy flow follows a specific sequence (figures 6-9 and 6-10). We can see that the Yang Connecting Extra Meridian carries within its width the overflow energies of the six Regular yin meridians. The Yin Connecting Extra Meridian carries the overflow energy of the six Regular yang meridians.

The Conception and Governor Vessels

Another interesting result of my exploration of the Extra Meridians was that,

Regular Meridian	Extra Meridian
Gallbladder	Conception
Liver	Governor
Stomach	Yin Connecting
Spleen	Yang Connecting
Triple Heater	Penetrating
Heart Constrictor	Belt
Large Intestine	Yin Connecting
Lung	Yang Connecting
Small Intestine	Yin Heel
Heart	Yang Heel
Bladder	Yin Heel
Kidney	Yang Heel

Figure 6-7 The Regular Meridians named on the left overflow into the Extra Meridians named on the right.

depending on whether my subject was male or female, I sensed, via the finger test, a difference in the direction of energy flow through the Conception and Governor vessels. As indicated in figure 6-7, the Liver Regular Meridian overflows into the Governor Vessel and the Gallbladder Regular Meridian overflows into the Conception Vessel. What I have found is that, in males, Liver energy flows up the Governor Vessel and Gallbladder energy flows down the Conception Vessel. Conversely, in females, Liver Meridian energy flows up the Conception Vessel and Gallbladder energy flows down the Governor Vessel. Thus it seems to me that the direction of energy flow in the Governor and Conception vessels is reversed for men and women. This leads me to further speculate that this may be why, on the TCM chart, both the Governor and Conception vessels are numbered sequentially from the bottom of the body. In other words, the chart makers based their illustration of the Conception Vessel on the female direction of energy flow, and their illustration of the Governor Vessel on that of males.

Tracing the Conception Vessel's flow in the area of the face and at the bottom of the feet drew my attention to another interesting phenomenon as illustrated in figure 6-11.

Ordinarily, the Conception Vessel's flow can be detected only in the areas indicated by solid lines; however, when the tongue is placed just behind the upper teeth at the top of the mouth, the energy flow is instantly detectable in the areas indicated by broken lines.

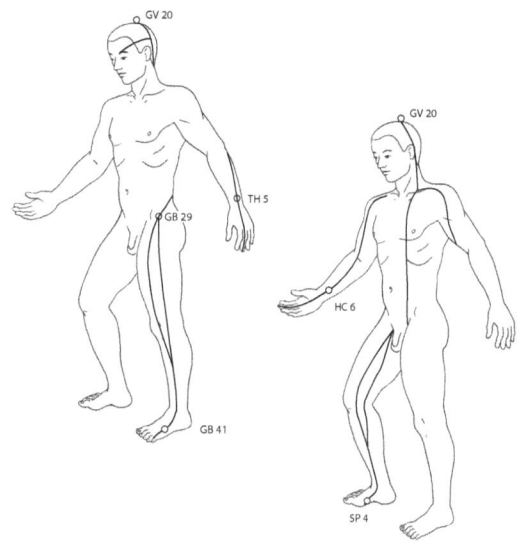

Figure 6-8 Yang Connecting and Yin Connecting Extra Meridians

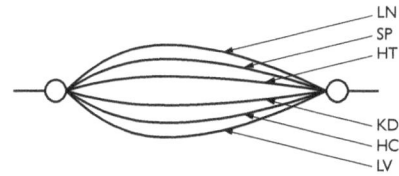

Figure 6-9 Yang Connecting Meridian (wide band)

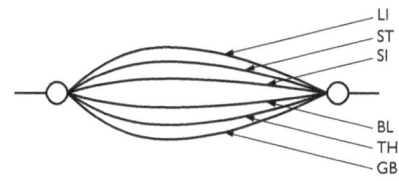

Figure 6-10 Yin Connecting Meridian (wide band)

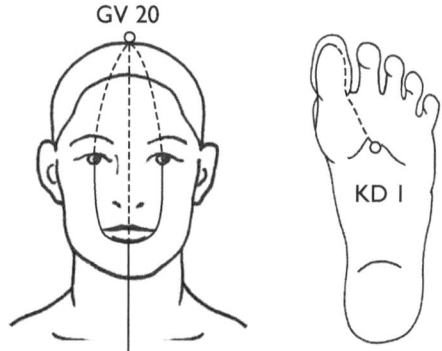

Figure 6-11 Conception Vessel flow in the area of the face and at the bottom of the feet

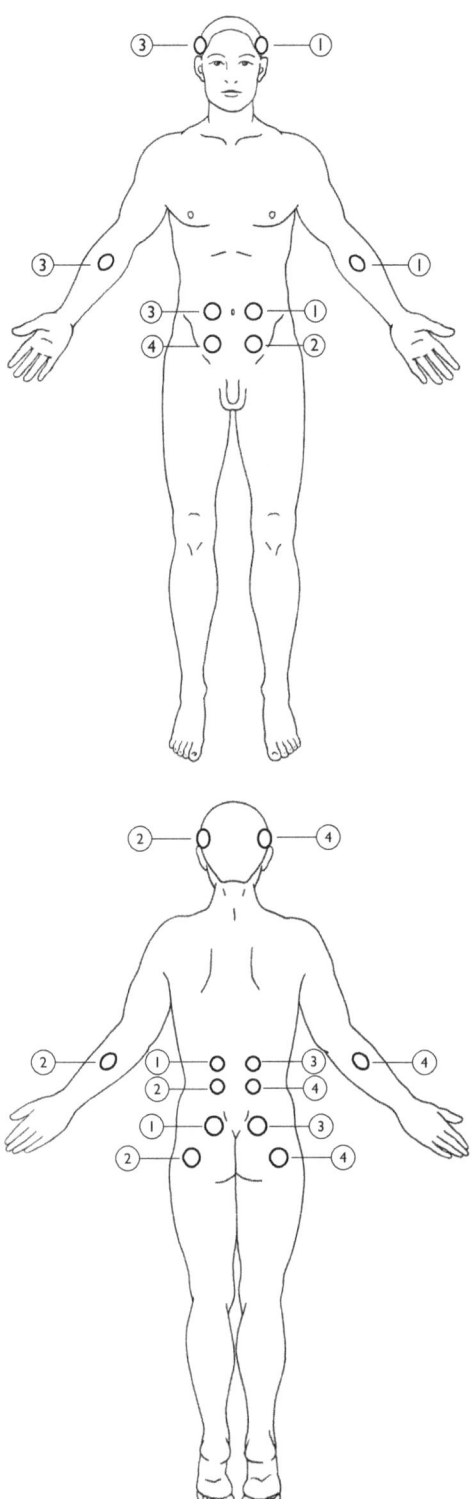

Figure 6-12 Extra Meridian energy circles are found at these locations on the body.

Extra Meridian Energy Circles

When the Extra Meridian system is called upon to regulate the Regular Meridian system, energy circles appear at certain locations on the body (see figure 6-12). (Refer to Chapter 2 for a more detailed description of the types and characteristics of energy circles.) I have found these energy circles to be of great use diagnostically, and they can be employed in treatment applications regarding the Extra Meridian system.

Each Extra Meridian energy circle is associated with two specific Extra Meridians as shown below.

Energy Circle 1 and 2	Conception/ Yin Heel Penetrating/Yin Connecting
Energy Circle 3 and 4	Governor/Yang Heel Belt/Yang Connecting

Figure 6-13 Energy Circles and the Extra Meridians associated with them

The energy circles appear on the body in numerical order, ascending with the degree of imbalance in the Extra Meridian system. When the Regular Meridians have just begun to spill over to the Extra Meridian system, the first energy circle appears. As the imbalance increases, circles 2 and 3 appear. When the imbalance is at its deepest level, the finger test will be positive for all four energy circles.

It is important to note that each energy circle is associated with a particular quality of Regular Meridian energy. As mentioned earlier, the yin Extra Meridians carry excess flow from the yang Regular Meridians, and the yang Extra Meridians carry the excess energy flow from the yin Regular Meridians. Energy circles 1 and 2 are associated with yin Extra Meridians. Thus the appearance of these two energy circles indicates trouble in one or more of the yang Regular Meridians. Energy circles 3 and 4 represent the yang Extra Meridians, and an imbalance in one or more of the yin Regular Meridians.

Energy circles appear at specific locations on the back, legs, arms and head, as detailed in figure 6-14.

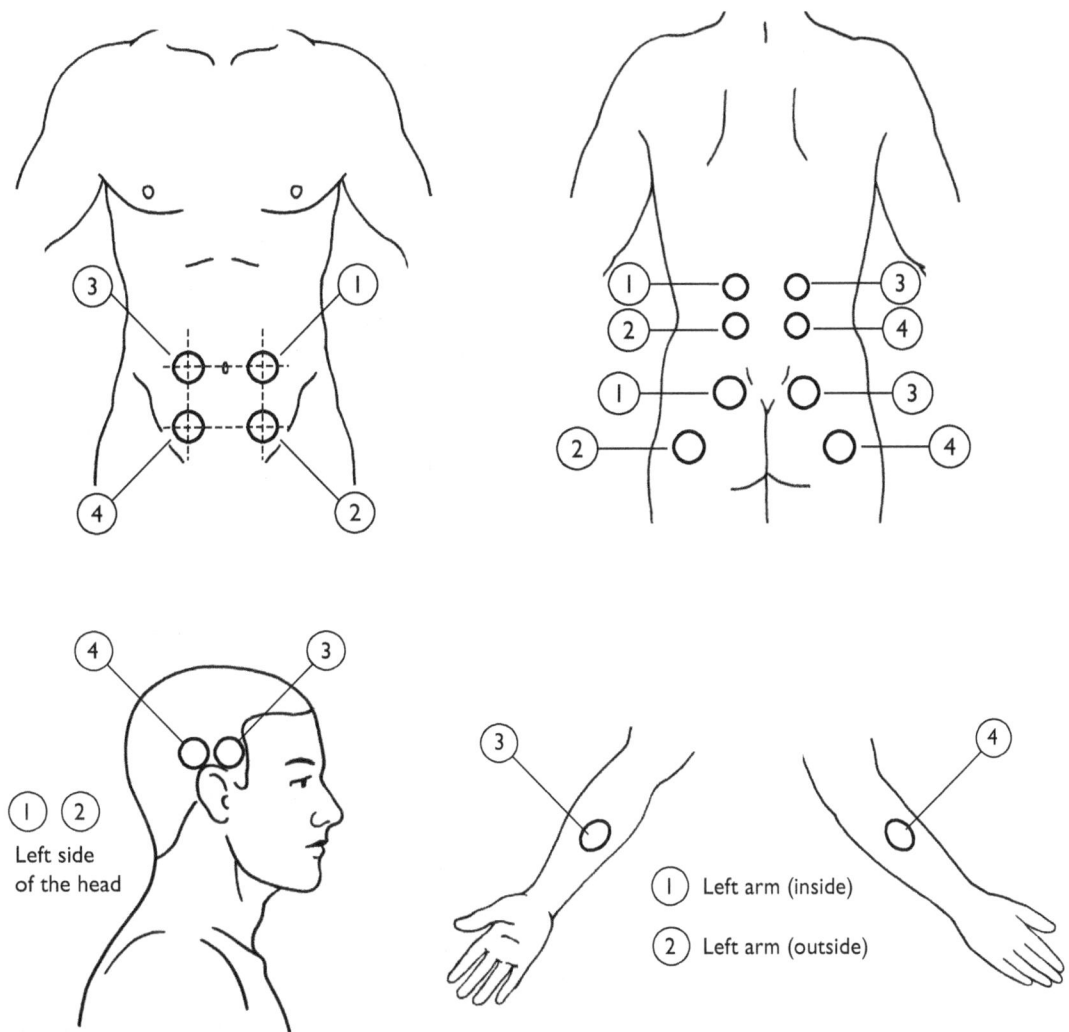

Figure 6-14 Close-up view of Extra Meridian energy circles

Extra Meridian Belt Zones

Another characteristic of the Extra Meridian system is the presence of belt zones on the legs and arms, similar to the Regular Meridian belt zones described in Chapter 2. Four zones corresponding to the yin Extra Meridians will be found on the arms; another four, corresponding to the yang Extra Meridians, will be found on the legs. Their width varies according to location: Extra Meridian belt zones on the arms are approximately 2 cun in width, while those on the leg are slightly wider, approximately 2.5 cun. See figure 6-15.

Sensing the Extra Meridians

With a good grounding in the Regular Meridian system and the Finger Test Method, one can skillfully sense and trace the Extra Meridians. This practice helps build an accurate working knowledge of the entire energy matrix and enhances our attunement to it. This in turn improves our diagnostic and treatment capabilities.

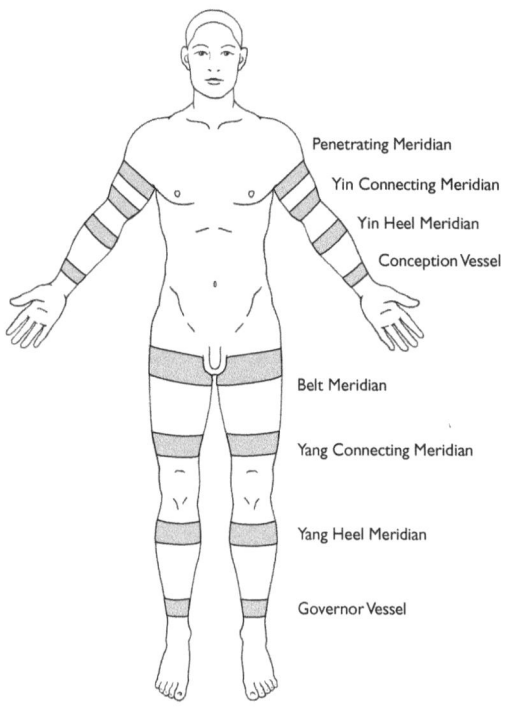

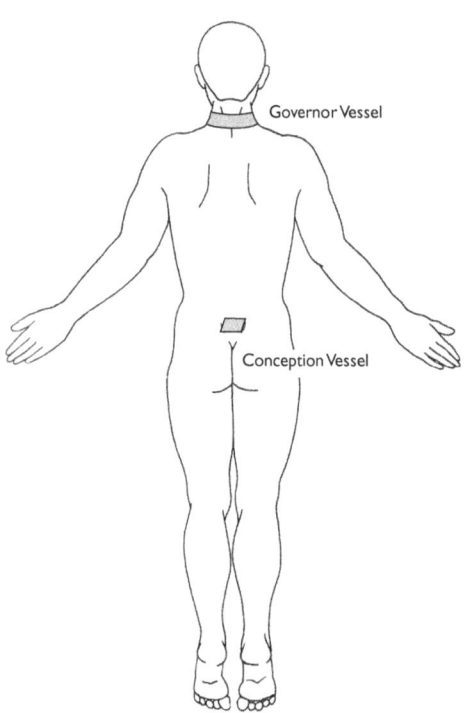

Figure 6-15 Extra Meridian belt zones

Extra Meridian Sound Images

Governor	Noh	Conception	Yu
Yang Heel	Shi	Yin Heel	Moh
Yang Connecting	Heh	Yin Connecting	Keh
Belt	Nu	Penetrating	Ru

Figure 6-16a Sound images for the Extra Meridians. Using these in conjunction with the Finger Test Method enhances our ability to detect the Extra Meridians. For more about sound imaging, see Chapter 3.

Instruction
Sensing the Extra Meridians

The Shin So Shiatsu method for locating the Extra Meridians is simple and effective. It is similar to Regular Meridian detection, except you must use:

- The Extra Meridian sensor.
- The sound image associated with each Extra Meridian (figure 6-16a).

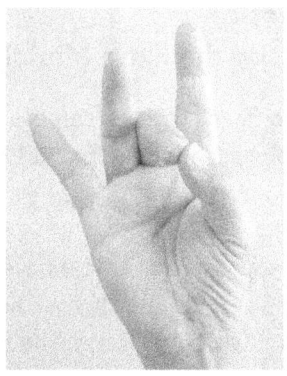

Figure 6-16b Extra Meridian sensor

It will be helpful to note that Extra Meridians are only one-third the width of Regular Meridians.

Instruction
Sensing Extra Meridian belt zones

By combining the finger test and sound imaging it is easy to find Extra Meridian belt zones.

1. Bring your Extra Meridian sensor toward the belt zone you are trying to locate. Use the general sensor only when the Extra Meridian zone in question is vibrating (see figure 6-18).

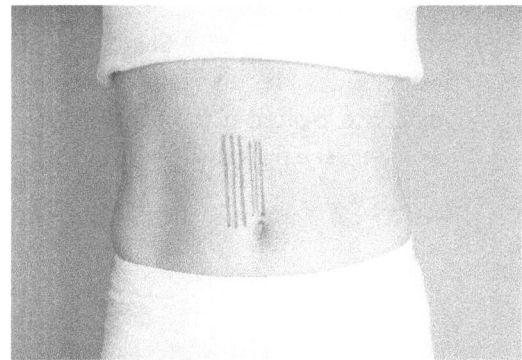

Figure 6-17 The Kidney Regular Meridian and Conception Vessel. Extra Meridians are one-third the width of Regular Meridians.

2. At the same time, image its corresponding sound, either audibly or silently. For example, if you wish to locate the Yin Heel Meridian belt zone on the arm, move your sensing hand down the length of the arm and image the sound "Moh."

When your sensor is above the belt zone for the Yin Heel Meridian your finger test will elicit a positive response. All Extra Meridian belt zones can be located using this technique.

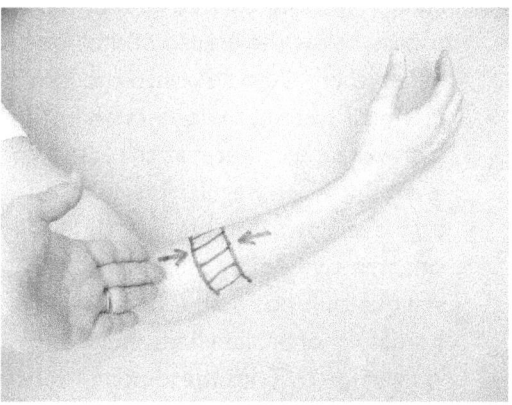

Figure 6-18 Sensing the Yin Heel Extra Meridian belt zone

Instruction
Diagnosing the Extra Meridians

With the finger test we can easily and accurately diagnose the Extra Meridian system.

1. Place your palm over the navel and image the sound "Zu." If your finger test elicits a sticky response, the Extra Meridian system is experiencing some degree of imbalance.

2. Confirm your diagnosis. Shin So Shiatsu Extra Meridian confirmation points are located at the back of the lower leg (see figure 6-19).

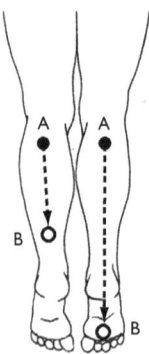

Figure 6-19 Shin So Shiatsu Extra Meridian confirmation points

Point A is located three to four finger widths below the crease of the knee. When there is no flow into the Extra Meridian system, the points on both legs will appear there, at the same level. But when Regular Meridian energy overflows into the Extra Meridians, the two points on the legs will start to shift position, following the trajectory of broken lines indicated in figure 6-19. Thus these points can be used to confirm whether or not the Extra Meridian system needs to be treated. To pinpoint their precise location, finger test along the back of the leg using your Extra Meridian sensor, and image the Extra Meridian associated sound "Zu." You will find that the two points will have moved downward, and to different locations on each leg.

3. Referring to figure 6-20, locate the four energy circles on the abdomen. Place your Extra Meridian sensor over the location of each circle and finger test to determine how many circles are vibrating.

Energy Circle 1 and 2	Conception/Yin Heel/Penetrating/Yin Connecting
Energy Circle 3 and 4	Governor/Yang Heel/Belt/Yang Connecting

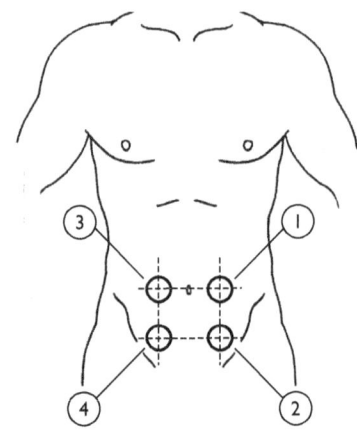

Figure 6-20 The four energy circles on the abdomen

4. If energy circles 1 or 2 elicit a sticky response, there is imbalance in the yin aspect of the Extra Meridian system. If energy circles 3 or 4 also elicit a sticky response, we know the yang aspect of the Extra Meridian system is out of balance.

5. Finally, we must determine which Extra Meridian is creating the disturbance in the system. For example, if energy circles 1 or 2 are vibrating, we know the problem lies in the yin Extra Meridians that traverse the leg medially. To diagnose which of these yin Extra Meridians needs treatment, scan your general sensor along the inside of the leg near the knee, and image the sound for each yin Extra Meridian. One sound only will elicit a sticky response and thus indicate which Extra Meridian needs treatment. If, for example, the sound "Moh" produces a sticky sensation, we know the Yin Heel meridian requires treatment. Refer to figure 6-21 and the sound image chart, figure 6-16.

6. If your sensor tells you energy circles 3 or 4 are active, you know the problem lies in the yang Extra meridians. In this case, you sweep your general sensor along the lateral aspect of the leg near the knee, while imaging the sounds associated with the yang Extra Meridians. The sound that elicits a sticky response corresponds to the particular yang meridian needing treatment.

7. You can also diagnose which Extra Meridian is out of balance by using the Extra Meridian belt zones described above. For example, if you sense that energy circles 1 and 2 are vibrating, place your Extra Meridian sensor two to three inches above each belt zone associated with those circles and image the question: in which zone is the Extra Meridian energy vibrating? The zone that elicits a sticky response corresponds to the Extra Meridian needing treatment.

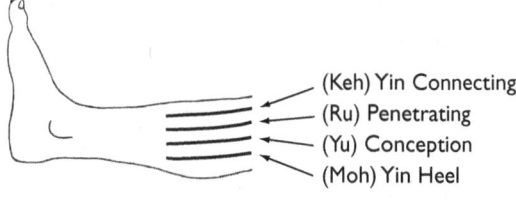

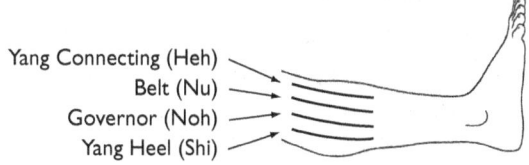

Figure 6-21 The yin and yang Extra Meridians as they flow along the medial and lateral aspects of the leg respectively

Treating the Extra Meridians

Despite renewed attention to Extra Meridians, relatively few acupuncturists work with them. There is even less discussion of this system among shiatsu therapists, though many of our patients experience imbalance at this deeper level. If we treat only the Regular Meridians, and perhaps achieve some balance there, the Extra Meridian system remains out of balance. And although the patient may feel some temporary relief, symptoms will not completely disappear and the original problem will once again fully manifest.

Extra Meridians can be the basis of either honji (foundational) or hyoji (target) treatments. Due to the jitsu nature of the energy they carry — energy that more closely reflects patient symptoms — a proper treatment can bring about quick relief, most notably for patients troubled by pelvic or other postural imbalances, muscle tension and spasms, and tendon problems. As already mentioned, a key function of the Extra Meridian system is to help the body cope with changes to its structural alignment.

And, although there is no direct connection between the Extra Meridians and the organs, Extra Meridian treatments do powerfully affect organ function. This is because, firstly, treating the Extra Meridian helps regulate the Regular Meridian system, which itself accesses and rebalances organ functions. But the Extra Meridians actually offer another more specific link with the organ functions of the Regular Meridians. For example, to treat the Belt and Yang Connecting Extra Meridians, we might choose to employ their Confluent Points (GB 41 and TH 5, see figure 6-2). These are yang Extra Meridians: we know they are handling overflow from the yin Regular Meridian system, and treating their Confluent Points would, of course, be useful in regulating the yin Regular Meridian system. It may even help regulate the Triple heater and Gallbladder Regular Meridians.

However, a complete treatment must also address the corresponding kyo imbalance (i.e. the more causative factor) or, again, our results will be short lived. As we shall explore further in the next chapter, the Divergent Meridian system receives the Regular Meridian system's overflow of kyo energy, and we will often find it is most appropriate to focus our treatment on the Divergent Meridians system. However, when we find an imbalance in the Extra Meridians, but not the Divergent Meridians, it is most prudent to treat the most kyo Regular Meridian.

Four main methods for treating Extra Meridian imbalances are detailed below:

- **Method 1**: Treating Extra Meridian energy circles using the yaki hari technique.

- **Method 2**: Treating Extra Meridians with shiatsu.

- **Method 3**: Treating Extra Meridians by removing ja ki.

- **Method 4**: Treating Extra Meridian Confluent Points with Ion Pumping (IP) cords.

Instruction — Method I
Energy circles and the yaki hari technique

I use the yaki hari method frequently in my practice. Yaki hari means "heated needle" in Japanese, but rather than needles, we use a small iron bar (figure 6-22d). We heat the bar to an effective but tolerable temperature using a lighter, then gently tap the surface of the patient's skin in a specific manner depending on our diagnosis of the energy circle we are treating.

Heat treatments such as moxibustion have a long history of use in Oriental medicine. The yaki hari approach I outline here was originally developed by Kurakichi Hirata (see "Hirata Zones," Chapter 2). Tadashi Irie later modified the technique to incorporate the iron bar. My own discovery of energy circles and the search for treatments to effectively balance the Extra Meridians led me to further refine the yaki hari method. I have found the results to be powerful and long lasting.

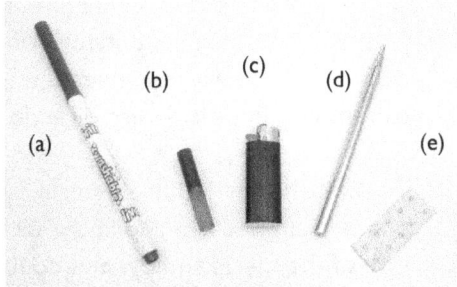

Figure 6-22 Yaki hari tools

a. Non-permanent marker
b. Bar magnet
c. Lighter
d. Small metal bar
e. Press tacks

Instruction — Method I
A. Diagnosing Extra Meridian energy circles

1. As soon as an Extra Meridian receives overflow from a Regular Meridian, one or more energy circles will begin to vibrate. Your first task is to ascertain how many energy circles are active. There will be as many as four vibrating circles, as illustrated in figure 6-12. Place your Extra Meridian sensor over each circle, starting with energy circle 1, and image the question: how many energy circles are active? The last energy circle you sense to be active is the one you treat. If you sense stickiness in energy circles 1, 2 and 3, treat energy circle 3, which reflects the system's deepest and most recent energy imbalance. When treated properly, the energy circles preceding it will automatically disappear.

2. Determine which group of energy circles (i.e. on the lower back, buttocks, abdomen, arms, or head) should be the focus of the yaki hari treatment. A simple rule is to follow the patient's main complaint: if it is located on the upper body, turn your attention to energy circles above the belt line; otherwise, use the energy circles on the hip.

3. Finger test to sense, then outline with a washable pen, the boundaries of the energy circle you need to treat.

4. Sense and draw three vertical and three horizontal energy lines within the circle. There are also six diagonal

lines, as shown in figure **6-23**, which are neither drawn nor diagnosed.

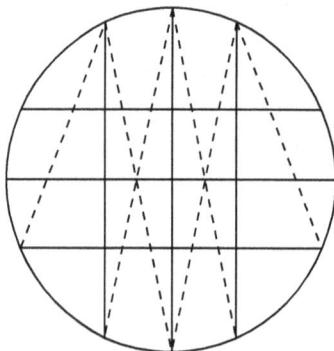

Figure 6-23 An energy circle

5. Determine whether the energy circle as a whole is kyo or jitsu in nature. Use the bar magnet: point the north pole (black end) down, towards the circle, and finger test. A sticky sensation tells you the energy circle is repelling the magnet's northern polarity (more tonifying than south-pole energy) and you can therefore assume the energy circle is jitsu in quality. To confirm, reverse the bar magnet, pointing the south pole (red end) towards the energy circle: a smooth sensation again tells you the energy circle is jitsu.

6. Determine the kyo or jitsu nature of each line you have drawn within the energy circle. Holding the magnet bar horizontally (with the black end pointing towards the patient's head when they are face down, and toward their feet when they are face up), diagnose each of the circle's three vertical lines. A smooth finger test result signifies the line is kyo; sticky signifies jitsu. Just one of the outer lines will be kyo; two will be jitsu (the middle vertical line is always jitsu). To remember which is which for your treatment, it helps to mark the kyo line.

7. To determine which horizontal lines in the energy circle are kyo or jitsu, position the magnet bar with the red end towards the patient's Governor Vessel, and follow the procedure as outlined above for diagnosing the vertical lines. Again, one of the outer lines will be kyo; and two will be jitsu (again, with the middle vertical line always jitsu).

Instruction – Method I
B. Treating Extra Meridian energy circles with yaki hari

1. Heat the metal bar to a comfortable temperature using the lighter and check with the patient to make sure it is not too hot.

2. If you have determined that the energy circle is jitsu in nature, gently and quickly double tap points demarcating the circle's outside borders, progressing in a counterclockwise direction. If the energy circle is kyo in nature, tap points demarcating its outside borders only once with the heated metal bar, moving in a clockwise direction.

3. To treat the vertical lines, single tap points along the kyo line in the direction of the meridian flow and double tap points along the jitsu line in the direction opposite the meridian flow.

4. To treat the horizontal lines, single tap points along the kyo line towards the Governor Vessel; double tap points along the jitsu line in the direc-

tion opposite the Governor Vessel's energy flow.

5. Sweep along the diagonal lines once from top to bottom.

6. To finish, place two press needles within the energy circles as indicated in figure 6-24. Place your palm gently over the energy circle for 15-20 seconds, allowing ja ki to release from the body.

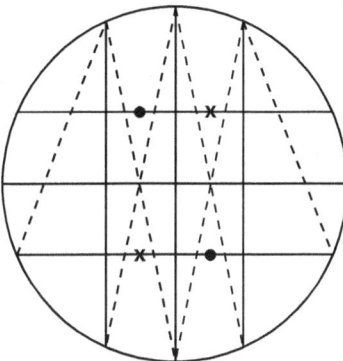

Figure 6-24 Two press needles are used, one on either side of the centre line, as shown.

Instruction – Method 1
C. Treating localized structural problems with yaki hari

The meridian system has the remarkable capacity to reveal not only purely energetic imbalances, but also to reveal, on the surface of the body, deeper structural issues affecting our patients. To localize structural imbalances causing joint, tendon, and muscle problems, we use the finger test in conjunction with sound imaging. I have found the most effective way to treat many neck, back, and shoulder problems is to perform the yaki hari protocol for structural problems as described below, and then, to follow it with the yaki hari treatment for Extra Meridian energy circles, described above.

1. Using your general sensor, scan the patient's body, or an area of their body, while imaging the sound "Neh." Use a marker or chopstick to better pinpoint the structural problem. A sticky response tells you where to focus your treatment.

2. Check the entire back and hip area for more energy circles that respond to the sound "Neh." When the imbalance is of a chronic or persistent nature, we will often find more than one energy circle vibrating. For example, an energy circle will often appear beside the thoracic region of the spine on the opposite side of an energy circle already identified in the sacral area. This is a result of muscular and structural compensation in the body.

3. At the focal point of the structural problem, sense and draw an energy circle: first its outside boundaries, then its vertical, horizontal, and diagonal meridian lines as described above.

4. Diagnose the circle and its lines, and treat it according to the protocol outlined above.

5. Follow with a yaki hari treatment of Extra Meridian energy circles.

Instruction – Method 1
D. Diagnosing and treating pelvic imbalances

The impact of Extra Meridian system imbalances on the body's structure is particularly evident in the pelvic region. When the Extra Meridians become activated, one side of the pelvis shifts upward, producing problems with the lower back and even the internal organs. A shift in the pelvis will affect the entire body: it can cause curvatures in the spine, unevenness in the legs, misalignments in the shoulders, neck, and skull. Extra Meridian treatments can help correct these and create the conditions for a deeper, long lasting change.

It is my observation that when energy circles 1 and 2 are vibrating, the left side of the pelvis is higher than the right. When energy circles 3 and 4 are activated, the reverse is true: the right side of the pelvis is higher than the left. See figure 6-25.

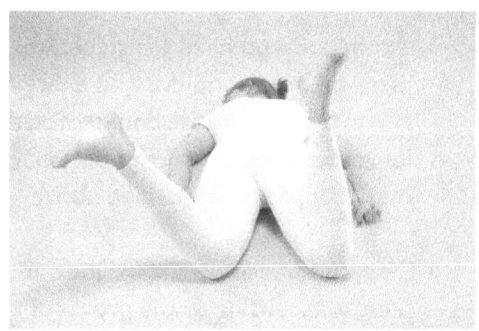

Figure 6-25 We will often find that particular shifts in the pelvis are reflected in the number of Extra Meridian energy circles vibrating.

1. After you have diagnosed the Extra Meridian energy circles, but before you proceed with your yaki hari treatment, ask your patient to lie face down. Grasp their legs at the ankles, and gently shake them to loosen the pelvic area. Bend their legs upward at the knees and support both lower legs at the ankles, allowing the feet to drop gently to either side. If energy circles 1 or 2 only are vibrating, the left leg will drop lower than the right. If energy circles 3 or 4 are vibrating, the right leg will drop lower than the left.

2. Perform your yaki hari treatment. Then, confirm the effectiveness of your treatment by re-checking the leg balance. Improvement is indicated by a more symmetrical positioning of the two legs (figure 6-26). (This method may not address pre-existing conditions such as structural damage to pelvic area and lower back through trauma.)

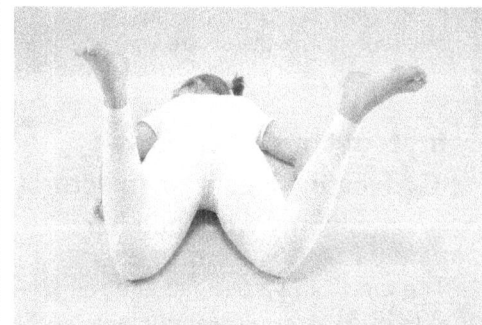

Figure 6-26 Legs are in a more symmetrical position after the yaki hari treatment.

Instruction – Method 2
Treating Extra Meridians with shiatsu

1. Ascertain which Extra Meridian needs support (and which Regular Meridian is overflowing into it). If for example, you find the Penetrating Extra Meridian

is being activated by an overflow from the Triple Heater Regular Meridian, you will also find energy circles 1 and 2 are vibrating (i.e. eliciting a sticky sensation with the finger test).

2. To treat this, with the patient face up, gently grasp their ankle with your hand in the Extra Meridian sensor position, and image the sound associated with the imbalanced Extra Meridian. In the case of the Penetrating Extra Meridian, you will image the sound "Ru." Slide the patient's foot upward until the finger test registers sticky. While maintaining that position at the hip, let the knee drop gently to the lateral side. See figures 6-27a and 6-27b. The Penetrating Meridian will begin to vibrate over the entire body.

3. When the leg is positioned correctly, energy circles 1 and 2 will disappear. Once you have confirmed this, precisely locate the Extra Meridian using the associated sound and general sensor. In this example, you treat the Penetrating Meridian where it flows along the medial side of the leg.

4. To correctly position the arm, refer to figure 6-28. When you are treating a yang Extra Meridian on the arm, the patient will be face down. When you are treating a yin Extra Meridian, the patient will be face up. Use the Extra Meridian sensor and the Extra Meridian sound image to position the arm. Use the general sensor and the Extra Meridian sound image to locate the meridian for treatment.

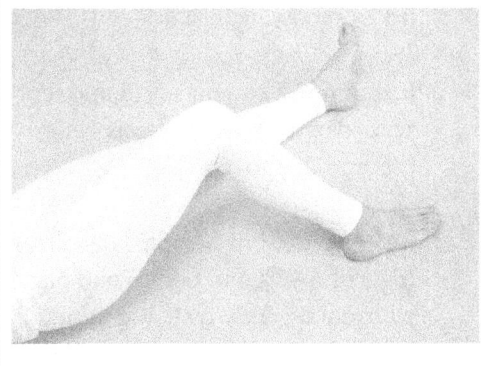

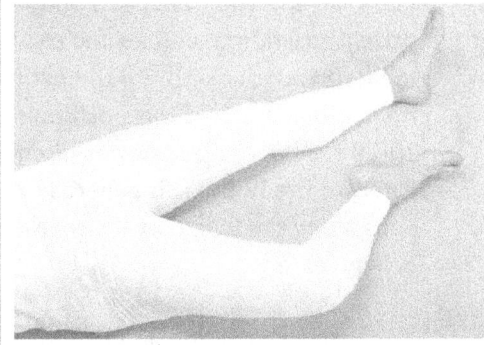

Figures 6-27a and 6-27b Open the patient's leg to the outside to access the Penetrating Meridian, the Extra Meridian associated with the Triple Heater Regular Meridian.

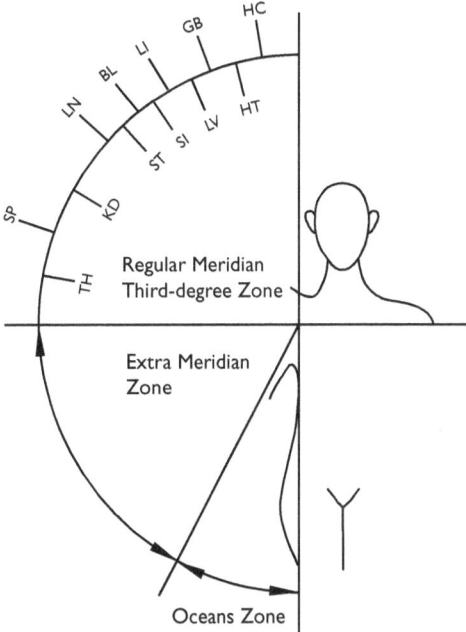

Figure 6-28 Arm positions for Extra Meridian shiatsu and ja ki removal treatments

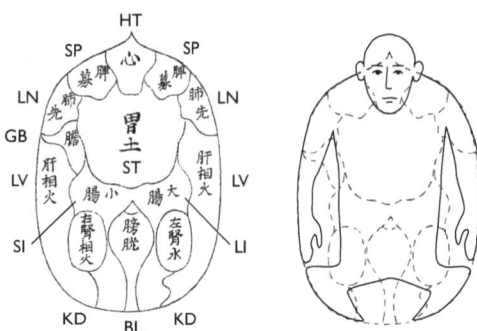

Figure 6-29a, 6-29b Mu Bun Sai Ja Ki charts (source: see *Reference Manual*, page 11)

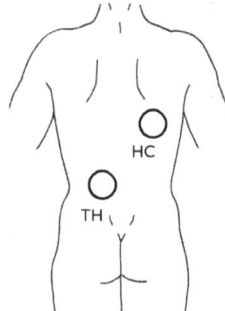

Figure 6-30 Shin So Shiatsu Ja Ki Chart

Note: The Mu Bun Sai Ja Ki Chart does not incorporate either the Heart Constrictor or Triple Heater Meridian zones: if your diagnosis calls for treatment of these, you must refer to this Shin So Shiatsu Ja Ki chart.

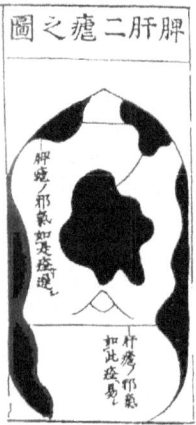

Figure 6-31 Ja ki chart drawn by the Buddhist monk Mu Bun Sai at an unknown date. The dark areas indicate ja ki present in the Liver and Spleen zones.

Instruction – Method 3
Treating Extra Meridians by removing ja ki

In cases where structural problems are most prevalent, treating Extra Meridian energy circles and the energy circles associated with structural imbalances provide the best results. But when it comes to mental/emotional problems or dysfunction in the organs, it is more effective to focus on removing ja ki from the meridians. With this type of treatment, the patient's energy remains in a state of balance for the longest possible duration, increasing chances of healing from these deeper, complex issues.

1. Ascertain which Extra Meridian is out of balance and the Regular Meridian overflowing into it.

2. Position the patient's arm and leg according to that diagnosis (as in Method 2, above).

3. Refer to the Mu Bun Sai Ja Ki Chart (figures 6-29a and 6-29b) and place your palm gently over the zone. For example, if you are treating the Spleen Meridian and you have positioned the patient's right arm and leg for treatment, place your palm on the patient's right shoulder. Hold this position for 10-20 seconds as ja ki begins discharging from the body. This generally happens along the length of the meridian being treated.

4. To sense the location and quantity of this ja ki emission, place your ja ki sensor four or five inches above the patient's body and image "A-o," the

sound used specifically for sensing ja ki. As long as ja ki is surfacing from deep inside the body, your finger test will elicit a sticky response. Once the process is complete, your finger test will register smooth.

5. Continue gently holding the patient's shoulder until you are confident that the ja ki has been completely eliminated. Repeat steps 2 and 3 on the opposite side of the body.

6. Complete the process of removing ja ki with the following three steps:

- remove ja ki from the spine;
- remove ja ki from the organs;
- apply palm pressure on the back.

a. Remove ja ki from the spine.
- Ask the patient to lie face down. Starting at the top of the spine, slide your palm gently down to the sacrum and finger test while imaging the question: where should I place my palms to continue facilitating the release of ja ki?
- Two areas usually elicit a sticky response. Place both palms gently on the patient's spine so that both palms are in contact with the areas you have identified. After 20-30 seconds, finger test to ensure ja ki is being released and then simply wait, with your hands off the patient, until you no longer sense ja ki releasing. Continue this process along the length of the spine.
- At the very bottom of the spine, in the area of coccyx, usually only one point tests positive for ja ki. Place both of your palms here, one on top of the other, and hold this point long enough to ensure that ja ki is removed from the end of the spine (usually 30-40 seconds).

b. Remove ja ki from the organs.
- For this process, refer to your Shin So back diagnostic chart.
- Place one palm on the sacrum and the other at the back of the head. Hold for about 30 seconds. Finger test to sense ja ki surfacing from the entire body. If necessary, you may repeat this process.
- Hold one palm on the patient's sacrum, shift the other hand from the patient's head to the first of up to three or four organ zones you prioritize for treatment. Your diagnosis may be based upon the following: what your patient tells you; your own sense there is a weakness in a particular organ or zone; the knowledge that your patient is experiencing a particular functional problem (such as with the stomach; in which case, you would place your palm on the Stomach diagnostic zone on the back).
- Repeat this process for each organ zone you wish to treat.

c. Palm pressure on the back.
- Place both palms on the patient's back and gently press areas where you sense ja ki is still surfacing.

7. Once you have successfully removed ja ki from the patient, the Extra and Regular meridians will be balanced. You can proceed with a general, whole body shiatsu treatment aimed at removing blockages, and paying special attention to the Shu Points on the back.

Instruction – Method 4
Treating Extra Meridian Confluent Points with ion pumping cords

This method is well documented in TCM literature and widely used by acupuncturists. Confluent Points, as shown in figures 6-32 and 6-33, serve to regulate Extra Meridians.

For example, Confluent Points GB 41 and TH 5 regulate the Belt and Yang Connecting meridians. These points are situated where the Yang Connecting Meridian and the Belt Meridian intersect. Shin So Shiatsu uses small aluminum posts instead of acupuncture needles. They are taped gently to the skin over the active Confluent Points, and IP cords are attached.

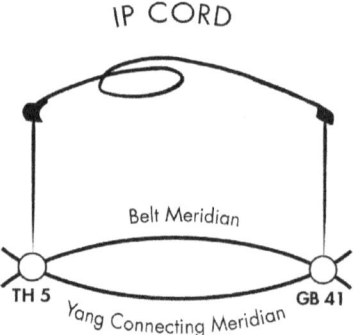

Figure 6-32 IP cord connecting two Confluent Points

1. To determine which Extra Meridian needs treatment, follow the approach outlined above in "diagnosing the Extra Meridians." You then use the Confluent Points for that meridian.

2. Confluent Points lie bilaterally on the body. You must choose the points on one side of the body or the other, which are active and most responsive to treatment. To determine this, use the imaging technique. Place your Extra Meridian sensor four to five inches above GB 41 on the left foot and then, above GB 41 on the right foot. Image the question: "which of these points is useful for treatment?" One point, GB 41 on either the right side or the left, will elicit a sticky sensation. This is the more effective treatment point. Use the same method to determine whether TH 5 on the right or left side is most useful for treatment. When you have ascertained this, tape the aluminum posts (or insert needles) onto GB 41 and TH 5 respectively.

3. Now determine which of these two points should be connected to the red (positive) or black (negative) clip on the ion pumping cord. Gently contact each aluminum post or acupuncture needle with one of the clips while performing the finger test. Attach the ion pumping cords to the post that elicits a sticky sensation. For example, if you contacted GB☐41 with the red clip, and finger tested sticky, attach the clip there. Now wait five to ten minutes.

4. To determine when the treatment is complete you again use sound imaging. Gently grasp the post or needle with your first-degree sensor and image the sound "Ji" while performing the finger test. "Ji" is the sound for diagnosing imbalances in the Regular Meridian system. Treating the Extra Meridians in this manner automatically addresses the Regular Meridians. When both treatment points test smooth, the treatment is finished.

Instruction
Locating acupuncture points using the Finger Test Method

1. Place your point sensor in the vicinity of the point you wish to locate.

2. Image the name of the point and finger test, moving your sensor in all directions until you get a sticky response.

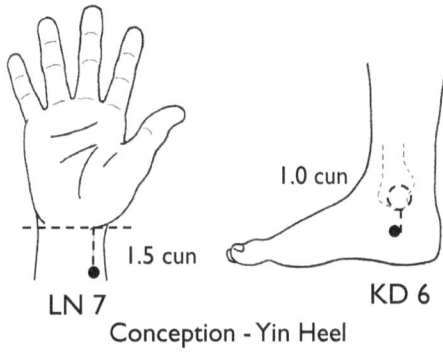
Conception - Yin Heel

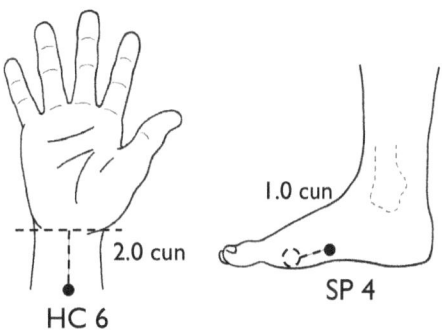
Yin connecting - Penetrating

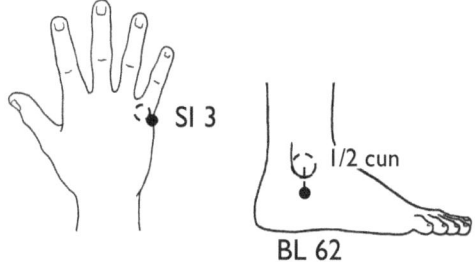
Governor - Yang Heel

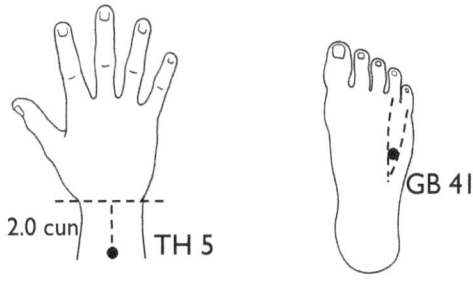
Yang Connecting - Belt

Figure 6-33 Confluent Points for Extra Meridian IP-cord treatment

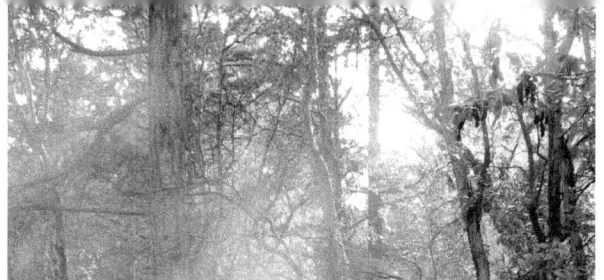

7

Diagnosing and Treating
The Divergent Meridians

the disused canal
what causes waves to rise
on the snow

- Shuoshi Mizuhara -

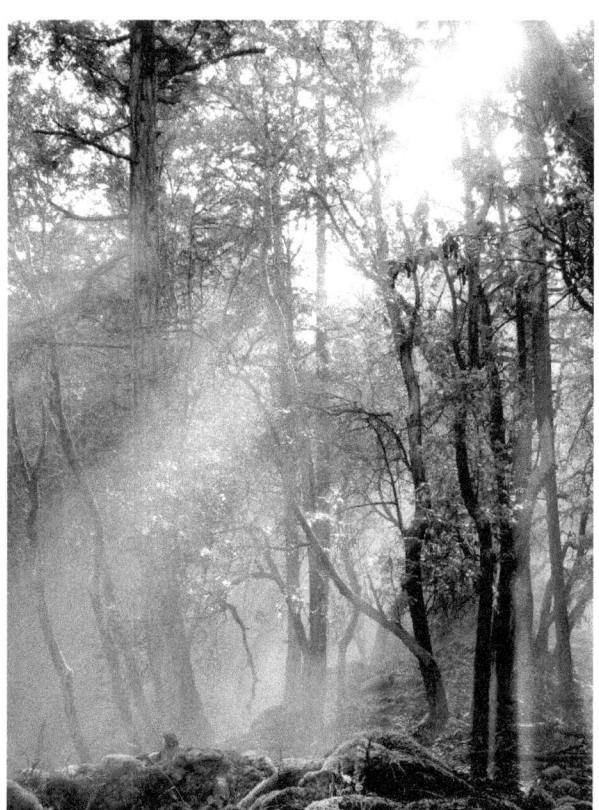

In this chapter, you will learn:

- How to distinguish Divergent Meridians from Regular and Extra Meridians.

- How to sense Divergent Meridians.

- How to diagnose a Divergent Meridian imbalance and confirm that diagnosis.

- How to find Divergent Meridian Crossing Points and Ratsu-ketsu Points, and use them in treatment.

- How to treat the Divergent Meridians using yaki hari, shiatsu, ja ki removal, and ion pumping methods.

Chapter 7

Diagnosing and Treating
The Divergent Meridians

When the Regular Meridians reach sho-sei-byo, their deepest level of disharmony, a sequence of changes takes place to help the body restore equilibrium. First, the Extra Meridian system is engaged. And if it cannot carry the Regular Meridian overflow, the Divergent Meridians are called into play. Most people will experience this level of imbalance from time to time; but for some, this energy state will be the norm. Whether it manifests briefly as a bad patch or endures as chronic illness, this is a critical juncture for treatment: yet many meridian therapists have never worked with the Divergent Meridians.

To be fair, the Divergent Meridians are considered an extension of the Regular Meridian system, and in contemporary annals, little is said about them. We know that their routes overlap with those of the Regular Meridians before they diverge, penetrating deeper into the body, bringing ki to the yin and yang organs. It is easy to speculate that a more refined understanding of this system could profoundly increase our capacity to harmonize organ functions — considered by many the central aim of Oriental medicine.

While Japanese acupuncturists have recently discovered — or rediscovered — this key component of our energetic physiology, the absence of detailed and accurate charts has hindered the duplication of research results and the development of treatment strategies. To develop my own working knowledge of this system and create a reliable foundation for further research, I set out to map precisely where and how the Divergent Meridians interconnect with the organs and other meridian systems. The diagnostic and treatment strategies that have flowed from this process have rendered some amazingly powerful results.

The TCM View

Following is a summary of our understanding of Divergent Meridians prior to my own research.

- The Divergent Meridians are an extension of the Regular Meridian system, but exist as an independent system or circuit, with their own locations and functions.

- Divergent Meridians function in pairs, as do Regular Meridians.

- Their primary function is to energetically link yin and yang organ pairs. The Kidney Divergent Meridian, for example, links the Kidney and Bladder. This link facilitates the "functional cooperation" between the two organs in a pair. For example, when one of a pair is weakened, the other may be similarly affected. In other cases, the opposite happens, and a weakened organ in a pair is shored up or strengthened by the other.

- There are 12 Divergent Meridians and they link the organs as illustrated in figure 7-1.

- Most, but not all, Divergent Meridians flow into the Heart organ.

- The general flow pattern for the Kidney/Bladder, Liver/Gallbladder, and Spleen/Stomach Divergent Meridian pairs is as follows. From the foot to the knee area, they overlap with their corresponding Regular Meridians. At the knee area, they penetrate deeper into the body, ultimately connecting with their corresponding organs. The meridian pairs meet at the face, head, or upper shoulder area.

- The general flow pattern for the Heart/Small Intestine, Heart Constrictor/Triple Heater and Lung/Large Intestine Divergent Meridian pairs is as follows. Flowing from the face, head, and shoulder area, they penetrate deeper into the body to connect with their corresponding organs. They then flow into the arm. Once they have reached the elbow area, they overlap with their corresponding Regular Meridian and flow more superficially along the forearm and into the hand.

Divergent Meridian	Linked Organs
Kidney	Kidney/Bladder
Bladder	Bladder/Kidney/Heart
Liver	Liver/Gallbladder/Heart
Gallbladder	Gallbladder/Liver/Heart
Spleen	Pancreas/Stomach/Heart
Stomach	Stomach/Pancreas/Heart
Heart	Heart/Small Intestine
Small Intestine	Small Intestine/Heart
Heart Constrictor	Heart/Triple Heater
Triple Heater	Triple Heater/Heart
Lung	Lung/Large Intestine/Heart
Large Intestine	Large Intestine/Lung/Heart

Figure 7-1 The Divergent Meridians and associated organs

Toward a More Complete Picture

Dr. Tadashi Irie made important contributions to Divergent Meridian research. His charts, presented below, provide an overview of his system's complete flow pattern.

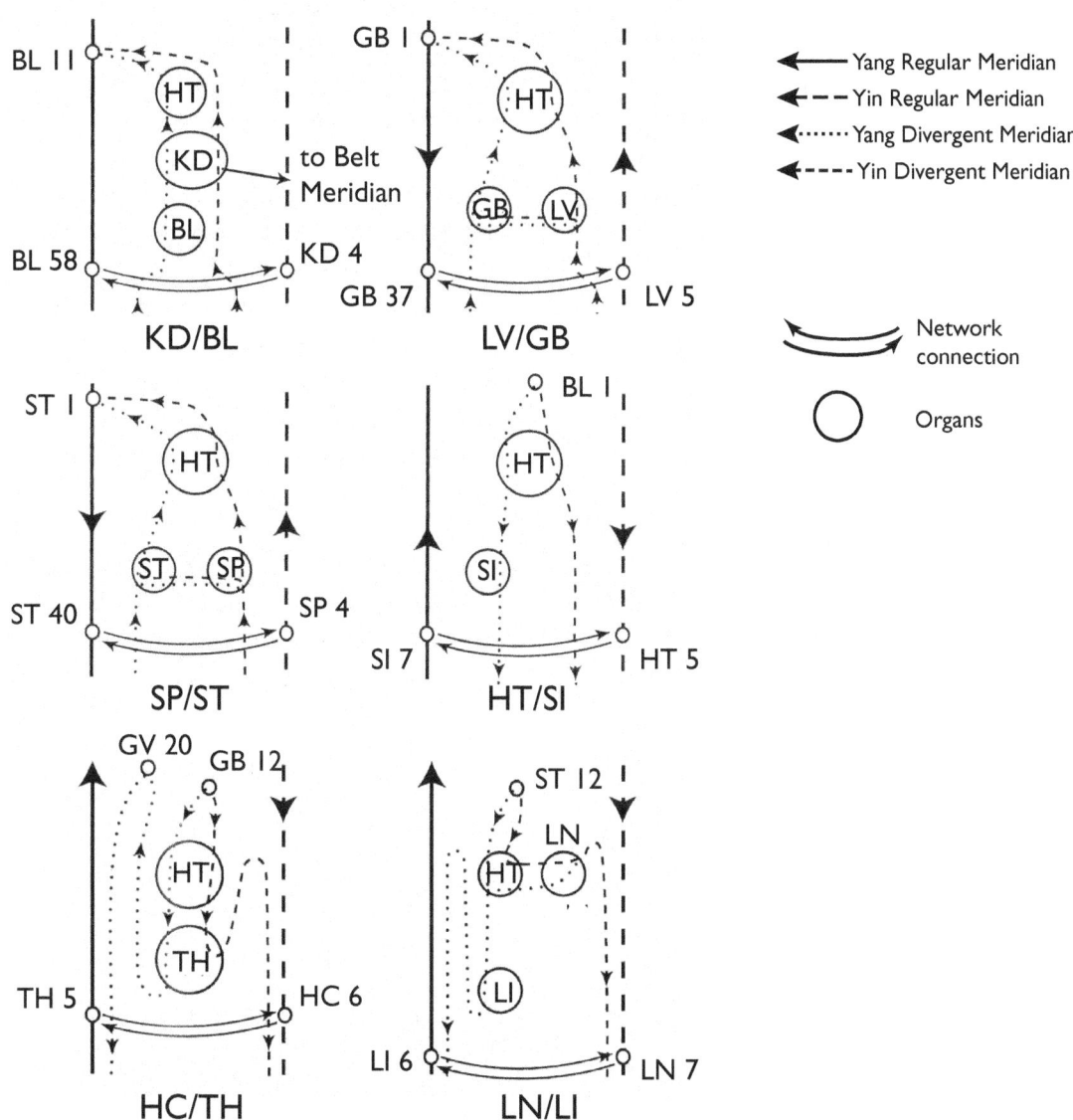

Figure 7-2 Dr. Tadashi Irie's Divergent Meridian charts (Ido No Nippon Sha, June 1981)

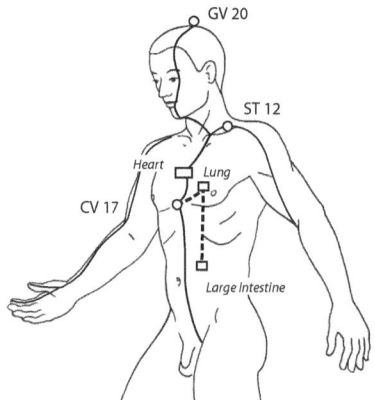

Figure 7-3a Lung Divergent Meridian

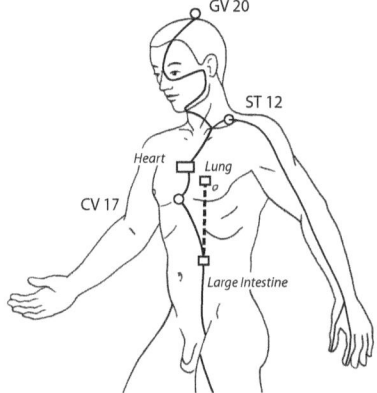

Figure 7-3b Large Intestine Divergent Meridian

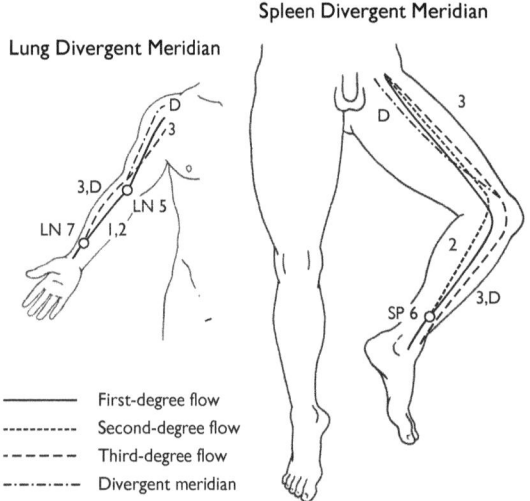

Figure 7-5 The Lung and Spleen Divergent Meridians as they appear on the lower arms and legs

Where They Flow:
The Divergent Meridians

My first task before tracing the intricate pathways of the Divergent Meridian system was to identify an effective finger test sensor (see figure 7-11). I found it among those developed by the renowned Japanese medical doctor and acupuncturist Dr. Hideo Yoshimoto, a respected member of the Irie Finger Test Group.

Once I had completed my own Divergent Meridian charts, I compared them with the prevailing TCM picture.

- The most notable difference in my charts was the presence of not one, but two distinctive branches of the Divergent Meridian system: one flowing superficially over the entire body; the second originating from specific points on the superficial pathway and penetrating deeper to the organs (see figures 7-3a and 7-3b).

- My research indicates that none of the Divergent Meridians flow into KD 1, as shown in figure 7-4: rather, the energy loops to the top of the foot.

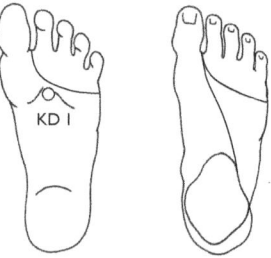

Figure 7-4 Large Intestine Divergent Meridian flow on the feet

- While TCM states most of the Divergent Meridians flow into the Heart organ, my research suggests they all do, via CV 17.

- My findings concur with TCM data which states that the Divergent Meridians overlap with the Regular Meridians on the lower arms and legs. However, my research suggests this overlapping occurs mostly along the Regular Meridian in its third degree (sho-sei-byo or organ disease level) of imbalance (see figure 7-5).

- All yin Divergent Meridians flow on the back of the body, into the coccyx area just above GV 1. Furthermore, they all flow along both sides of the spine, and overlap with one another (see figure 7-6).

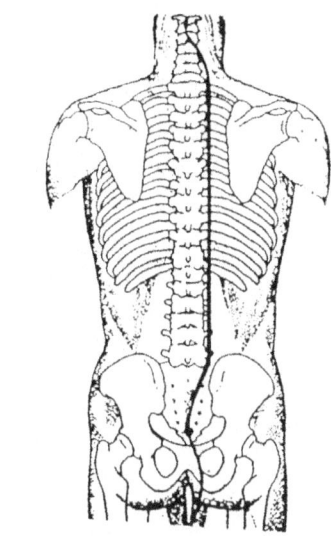

Figure 7-6 Divergent Meridians flow along the spine.

Further Findings

The finger test helped me fine-tune my understanding, appreciation, and working knowledge of the Divergent Meridians. I learned the following:

- In the head, face, and upper neck area, when a yang Divergent Meridian is balanced, we will be able to sense its flow along the entire pathway, as indicated by the solid and dotted lines. If a particular Divergent Meridian is in a state of imbalance, however, we will not be able to sense its flow along the section of the pathway indicated by the dotted line. With successful treatment of the imbalance, it will again be possible to detect the flow of energy along the entire pathway. It appears that, by treating the Divergent Meridian, the energy will more completely fill its pathways and thus flow as one connected channel. Figure 7-7 illustrates this interesting phenomenon in Divergent Meridian flow.

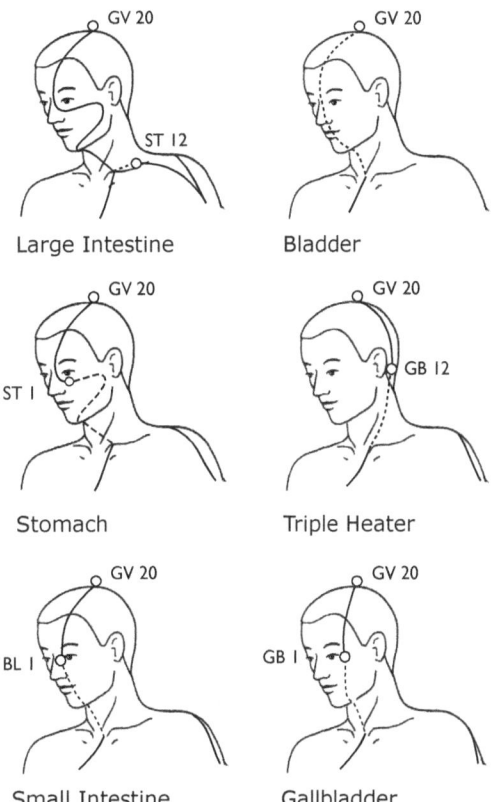

Figure 7-7 When a yang Divergent Meridian is out of balance, we are unable to sense its flow along the pathway as indicated by a dotted line.

- The yin Divergent Meridians manifest a phenomenon similar to the one described above. The yin Divergent Meridians all flow into the cervical region of the spine, overlap with the Governor Meridian, and continue up to GV 20. However, if any of the yin or yang Divergent Meridians are out of balance, we will not be able to detect their energy flow between the cervical area and the top of the head at GV 20. Figure 7-8 illustrates this.

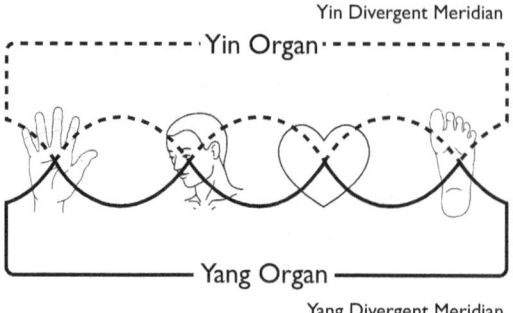

Figure 7-9 Intersection points for Divergent Meridian pairs

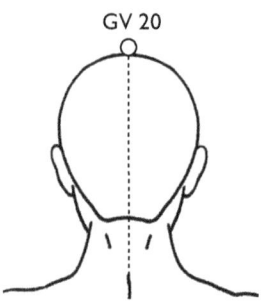

Figure 7-8 When a yin Divergent Meridian is out of balance, we are unable to sense its flow along the pathway indicated by a dotted line.

Crossing Points and Ratsu-ketsu Points

Each Divergent Meridian pair intersects at four areas of the body: the lower arm, lower leg, face and upper back, and heart area (figure 7-9). At these intersections, TCM has identified treatment points — referred to as Crossing Points — for the Divergent Meridian system. My own research confirms the existence of these very effective points: they are described in more detail later, under "treating Divergent Meridians with IP cords."

Another important category of treatment points — Ratsu-ketsu Points (connecting acupuncture points) — are located along the short pathways which bridge the paired Divergent Meridians. These bridges occur at particular locations, such as the wrist and ankle areas, and can be clearly detected using the Divergent meridian sensor and the sound image for the associated Regular Meridian. One such bridge, for example, links the Lung and Large Intestine Divergent meridians at Ratsu-ketsu Points LN 7 and LI 6 (figure 7-10). Ratsu-ketsu Points are also discussed under "treating Divergent Meridians with IP cords."

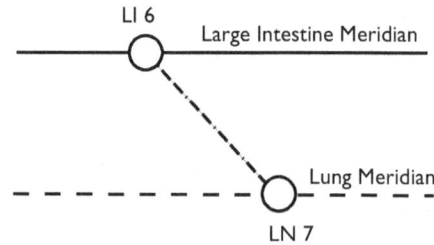

Figure 7-10 Ratsu-ketsu Points

Diagnosing the Divergent Meridians

Because the Divergent Meridian system is an extension of the Regular Meridian system, we can diagnose it using either the Regular Meridian abdominal chart for the third degree or the Back Diagnostic Chart. We must, however, use the Divergent Meridian sensor (figure 7-11).

Instruction
Diagnosing the Divergent Meridians

1. To determine whether the Divergent Meridian system is out of balance, place your general sensor five to six inches above the patient's navel area. Perform the finger test while imaging the sound "De." A sticky response tells you there is an imbalance in this system.

2. To confirm your answer, place your Divergent sensor at the back of the patient's head. All yin Divergent Meridians overlap here with the Governor Meridian. Image the name of any Regular Meridian and finger test. A smooth response indicates the Divergent Meridian system is out of balance (see figure 7-12).

3. Refer to the back diagnostic chart in your *Reference Manual* to determine which of the Divergent Meridians is out of balance. Hold your Divergent Meridian sensor one to two inches above the patient's spine and perform the finger test, imaging the sound "De." Move your sensor down the spine from the first thoracic vertebra to the sacrum. Remember that if you detect stickiness in the zones located between T7 and T9, you must now decide which of the four possible meridian zones here are active: the Heart Constrictor, Stomach, Liver, or Gallbladder.

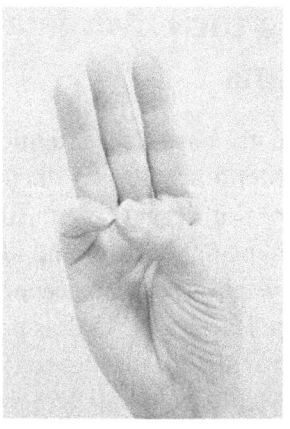

Figure 7-11 Divergent Meridian sensor

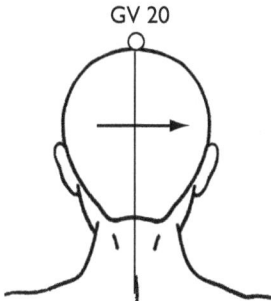

Figure 7-12 Confirming a Divergent Meridian imbalance

Treating the Divergent Meridians

Shin So Shiatsu pays close attention to the Divergent Meridians. Proper diagnosis and treatment of this deeper system simultaneously rebalances the Extra and Regular Meridian system — at first, second, and third degree levels. The result is powerful.

The four main approaches to treating Divergent Meridian imbalances are:

- **Method 1:** Treating Divergent Meridian energy circles with the yaki hari technique.

- **Method 2:** Treating Divergent Meridians with shiatsu.

- **Method 3:** Treating Divergent Meridians by removing ja ki.

- **Method 4:** Treating Divergent Meridians with IP cords.

Instruction — Method 1
Treating the Divergent Meridians with the yaki hari technique

The yaki hari technique is one of my favourite methods for treating the Divergent Meridian system. It's fast and efficient, and the benefits last. Two approaches are described below. I recommend you become familiar with the first, more basic method, before moving on to the second one.

A. Basic yaki hari treatment

1. Once you know the patient requires treatment at the Divergent Meridian level, identify which meridian you should focus on, as described above.

2. Find the energy circle associated with the out-of-balance Divergent Meridian (for a review of energy circles, see chapters 2 and 6). This energy circle may appear on either side of the spine and will be located at approximately the same vertebral level as the Regular Meridian Back Shu Point (for Shu Points, see *Reference Manual*). For example, the Liver Divergent Meridian energy circle will be near T10 and the Liver Shu Point (see *Reference Manual*). Hold your Divergent Meridian sensor an inch or two from the patient's spine on one side or the other; image the meridian name as you scan from the first thoracic vertebrae down to the coccyx. When your sensor reaches the energy circle in need of treatment, the finger test will read sticky. (If you don't find the circle on the first side of the spine, check the other side.)

3. Hold your pen with the Divergent Meridian sensor, image the meridian name, and trace out the energy circle.

4. Draw the meridian lines inside the circle, then diagnose the circle and lines as we did with Extra Meridian circles.

5. Treat the circle according to the instructions given for the Extra Meridians. (See Chapter 6).

B. Advanced yaki hari treatment

Whenever the Divergent Meridian system is out of balance, we will find the Extra Meridian system is also out of balance. The kyo energy of the Regular Meridians overflows into the Divergent Meridians; jitsu energy overflows into the Extra Meridians. In treating the Divergent Meridian system, we are dealing with the root of the problem. Working with the Extra Meridians addresses symptoms that arise due to this imbalance. By treating both systems, we can expect a better result than by treating just the Divergent Meridians.

As explained above, all 12 Divergent Meridians flow into the Heart organ via CV 17 (see figure 7-13). It is relatively easy to sense the Divergent Meridians here.

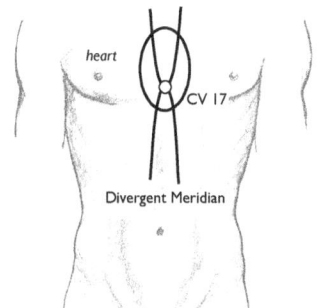

Figure 7-13

1. Place your Divergent Meridian sensor at CV 17 (Position A on figure 7-14): one by one, image the names of the 12 Divergent Meridians. Note: When a Divergent Meridian's energy is in a balanced state, we experience a *sticky* sensation here when imaging its name. When a meridian requires treatment, we get a *smooth* response.

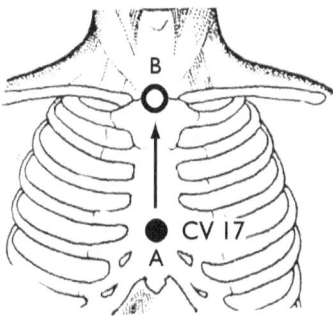

Figure 7-14 Divergent Meridian confirmation point

2. Now image the name of the meridian needing treatment, and while doing so, move your Divergent Meridian sensor along the sternum towards the patient's head.

3. One point along the sternum will test sticky. The farther up the sternum you find this point, the greater the imbalance being reflected in that particular meridian.

As stated, when a Divergent Meridian is out of balance to any degree, finger testing while imaging its name will result in a *smooth* response at Position A (in figure 7-14). You will get a *sticky* response for that meridian somewhere between positions A and B (just below CV 22).

If the sticky response does not come until you have reached the uppermost position (at B) it means the Divergent Meridian in question is fully out of balance. When this happens, you will be also able to detect this same out-of-balance Divergent Meridian in the back diagnostic area (or in the front third-degree zone), using your Divergent Meridian sensor.

As well, when you test over the abdomen using the sound image "De," you will receive a positive result, indicating that the overall body imbalance has fully engaged the Divergent Meridian system.

However, when you find the sticky response somewhere between position A and B, you will not normally detect the imbalanced meridian in the back or front diagnostic area, nor will testing with the "De" sound over the abdomen yield a positive result. In this case, you are working with a "hidden" Divergent Meridian.

A hidden Divergent Meridian indicates a growing imbalance — that a Divergent Meridian is engaged in receiving kyo energy from a third-degree Regular Meridian, but that it is not yet overwhelmed by it. It is thus very much indicated for treatment, and can be addressed by the yaki hari technique. However, the Divergent Meridian energy circle may appear anywhere on the back, rather than only in the area of the Back Shu Point for that organ function.

To recap, then: when a Divergent Meridian is not fully out of balance, i.e. eliciting a sticky response somewhere between positions A and B, and not detectable along the spine, you can still treat it using the yaki hari technique. But in this case, you must look for the energy circle not only in the area of the Back Shu Point but anywhere on the back.

4. Locate the Divergent Meridian energy circle on the back using your Divergent Meridian sensor and imaging the name of the imbalanced meridian. Follow the basic approach outlined above to draw and diagnose this circle.

5. Refer back to your initial diagnosis of the Extra Meridian system: locate, diagnose, and treat the vibrating Extra Meridian circle. If the patient's main problem area is above the waist, treat the circle on the lower back; if it is below the waist, treat the circle in the hip area.

6. Finally, treat the Divergent Meridian energy circle.

Instruction — Method 2
Treating the Divergent Meridians with shiatsu

The method for treating Divergent Meridians with shiatsu is essentially the same as our method for treating the most kyo-most jitsu Regular Meridians described in Chapter 5. The only difference is the bending positions for the legs and arms.

1. To find the correct bending position for the Divergent Meridian you are treating, adopt the Divergent Meridian sensor position, gently grasp the patient's leg near the ankle, and image the name of the meridian you are seeking. Slide the patient's foot up or down to the position that elicits a

sticky sensation. Refer to the Divergent Meridian belt zone chart (figure 7-15) for more help in locating the correct treatment position.

2. We use the same method to position the arm for a Divergent Meridian treatment. Again, with your hand in the Divergent Meridian sensor position, image the name of the meridian needing treatment, and hold the patient's arm at the wrist. Gently slide the arm within the Divergent Meridian zone (see figure 7-16) until the finger test elicits a sticky response.

Instruction — Method 3
Treating the Divergent Meridians by removing ja ki

When a patient's ki is chronically out of balance at the Divergent Meridian level, it may be necessary to remove ja ki at a deeper energetic level to see a noticeable improvement.

1. Begin as you would to treat the Divergent Meridians with shiatsu (Method 2). Diagnose which Divergent Meridian is out of balance. Position the patient's leg according to figure 7-15. To confirm that you have the correct bending position, place your Divergent Meridian sensor over Position B (at the top of the sternum as shown in figure 7-14) and finger test: a smooth response says your placement is correct.

   For example, if the Liver Divergent Meridian is fully out of balance, you will get a sticky response when you finger test for it at Position B. But when you position the patient's

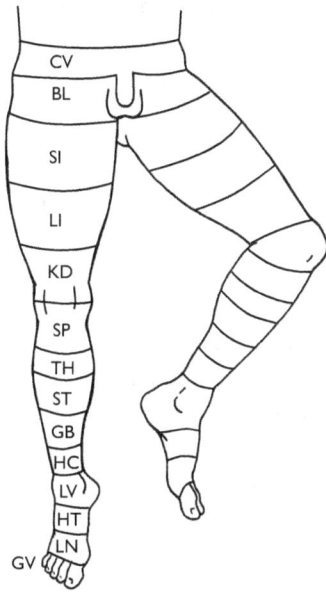

Figure 7-15 Divergent Meridian belt zones for positioning leg

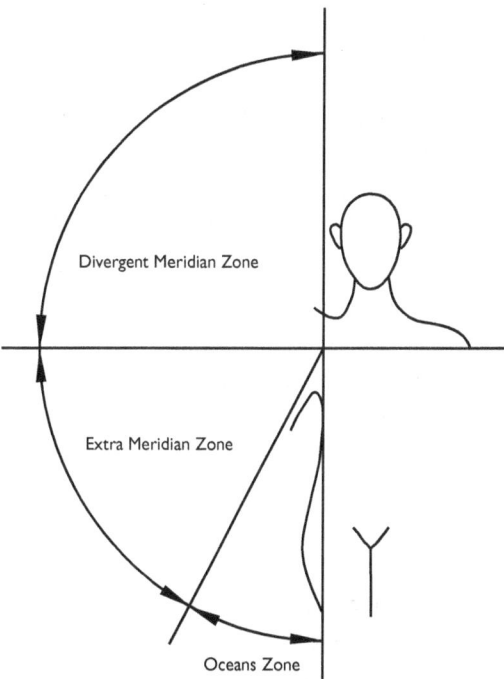

Figure 7-16 Arm positions for treating the Divergent Meridians

leg according to the chart and finger test at Position B again, you will get a smooth response.

2. Next, using the finger test and figure 7-16 to guide you, position the arm to activate the Liver Divergent Meridian on the same side as you did the leg. To confirm that you have done this accurately, place your Divergent Meridian sensor over Position B, image the name "Liver Meridian," and finger test. This time, you should get a sticky response.

3. With the leg and arm correctly placed, refer to your Mu Bun Sai Ja Ki Chart (figures **6-29**, **6-30**, and *Reference Manual*): gently place your palm on the area(s) of the patient's body associated on the chart with the Liver Meridian. Finger testing while imaging the sound "A-o" will tell you when ja ki has begun to release from along the length of this Divergent Meridian (within about 10-15 seconds). Continue monitoring release of ja ki until you can no longer sense it (this may take several minutes). Carry out the same process on the opposite side of the body.

4. Ask the patient to lie face down. Starting at the top of their head, slide your palm gently along their spine to the sacrum and finger test while imaging the question: where should I place my palms to continue facilitating the release of ja ki? One or two areas usually elicit a sticky response. Place both palms gently on the patient's back, so that one or both are in contact with the areas you have identified. After 10-15 seconds, finger test to ensure ja ki is being released and then, simply wait, with your hands off the patient, until you no longer sense ja ki releasing. Continue this process along the length of the spine, above and below your starting points, placing your palms, triggering the release of ja ki, and monitoring its release with your hands off the patient.

5. The Divergent Meridian system should now be balanced. Follow with a whole-body shiatsu treatment to eliminate muscular tension. Ensure you do not over stimulate the patient: 30 minutes should be sufficient.

Instruction — Method 4
Treating the Divergent Meridians with IP cords

This is a very effective method for realigning the body's deeper energies. It is similar to that described in Chapter 6 for treating the Extra Meridian system. In that case, we connected IP cords to Extra Meridian Confluent Points.

Here, we treat points situated where the paired Divergent Meridians meet (Divergent Meridian Crossing Points) and Ratsu-ketsu Points. One point is always chosen from the face or upper body area. The second point will be found on the arm or the leg, depending on the Divergent Meridian you are treating.

Ratsu-ketsu Points for the Lung, Large Intestine, Heart Constrictor, Triple Heater, Heart, and Small Intestine Divergent Meridians are on the lower arm.

Ratsu-ketsu Points for the Spleen, Stomach, Liver, Gallbladder, Kidney, and

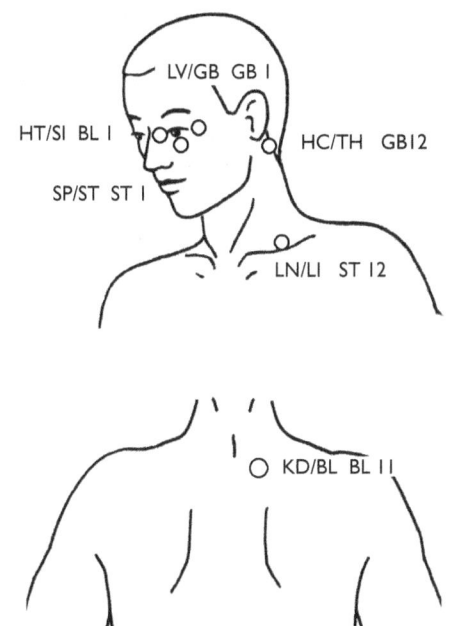

Figure 7-17a Divergent Meridian Crossing Points on the face and upper body

Divergent Meridian Pair	Crossing Point
Lung/Large Intestine	ST 12
Spleen/Stomach	ST 1
Heart/Small Intestine	BL 1
Kidney/Bladder	BL 11
Heart Constrictor/Triple Heater	GB 12
Liver/Gallbladder	GB 1

Figure 7-17b

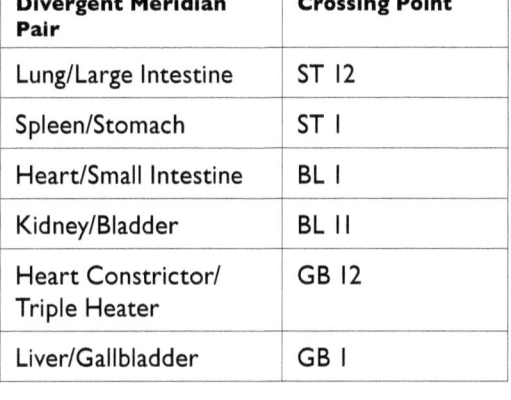

Figure 7-18a Ratsu-ketsu Points on the arms

Arm Meridian	Ratsu-ketsu Point
Lung	LN 7
Large Intestine	LI 6
Heart Constrictor	HC 6
Triple Heater	TH 5
Heart	HT 5
Small Intestine	SI 7

Figure 7-18b

Figure 7-19a Ratsu-ketsu Points on the legs

Leg Meridian	Ratsu-ketsu Point
Spleen	SP 4
Stomach	ST 40
Liver	LV 5
Gallbladder	GB 37
Kidney	KD 4
Bladder	BL 58

Figure 7-19b

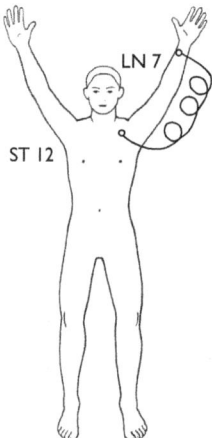

Figure 7-20 IP cord hook-up sequence for the Lung Divergent Meridian. The Ratsu-ketsu Point for the Lung Divergent Meridian is LN 7. It is paired with a Crossing Point on the face or upper body, in this case, ST 12.

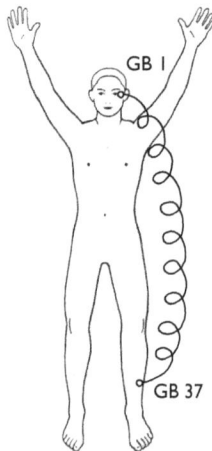

Figure 7-21 IP cord hook-up sequence for the Gallbladder Divergent Meridian. Here, the Ratsu-ketsu Point GB 37 is paired with GB 1, the Gallbladder Divergent Meridian Crossing Point.

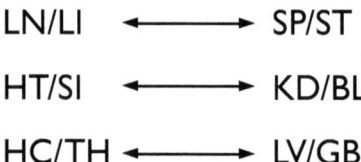

Figure 7-22 Two Divergent Meridians are treated with IP cords. When the meridians on the left are imbalanced, they are treated in conjunction with those shown on the right, and vice versa.

Bladder Divergent Meridians are on the lower leg.

By attaching only one IP cord to the patient, we regulate only half the body. To treat the whole body, we need a second IP cord. Figure 7-22 illustrates which Divergent Meridians should be treated in addition to the one initially diagnosed for treatment. For example, if the Lung Divergent Meridian requires treatment, the chart indicates you would also treat the Spleen Divergent Meridian with an IP cord. This two-cord system was developed by Dr. Tadashi Irie.

To treat the Lung/Large Intestine, Heart Constrictor/Triple Heater, or Heart/Small Intestine Divergent Meridians, affix a second IP cord to the opposite side of the body.

For the Spleen/Stomach, Liver/Gallbladder, and Kidney/Bladder Divergent Meridians, the second cord will be on the same side of the body as the first.

Instruction — Method 4
Executing the IP cord protocol

1. Determine which Divergent Meridian should be treated.

2. Accurately locate the Divergent Meridian treatment points for that meridian. For example, if you have diagnosed imbalance in the Lung Divergent Meridian, you will be looking for the Lung/Large Intestine Crossing Point, ST 12, and the Ratsu-ketsu Point, LN 7. To enhance accuracy, hold a chopstick or a pencil between your thumb and little finger (the Divergent Meridian sensor position). When your sensor meets the correct point for the meridian pair, it will elicit a sticky sensation.

3. Determine which side of the body should be treated: i.e. should the IP cord be affixed to ST 12 and LN 7 on the right side or the left? Hold your Divergent Meridian sensor about eight inches over ST 12 on the right side and then on the left. Image the question: which point is most suitable for treatment? One will read sticky, one smooth. Treat the smooth one.

4. Tape aluminium posts to (or insert acupuncture needles into) the two points you have selected.

5. You must now determine which of these two points should be connected to the red (positive) clip on the IP cord and which one should be connected to the black (negative) clip. Gently contact each post or acupuncture needle with one of the clips while performing the finger test. Attach the IP cord to the point that elicits a smooth sensation.

6. Finally, affix the second IP cord to the opposite side of the body, in this case, at SP 4 and ST 1.

7. Divergent Meridian treatments regulate the Divergent, Extra, and Regular Meridians. To determine if your treatment is complete, place your palm above the patient's tanden and image the sound "Ji." When the finger test begins to elicit a smooth sensation, the treatment is complete. To solidify the treatment gains, keep the IP cords attached for another five minutes.

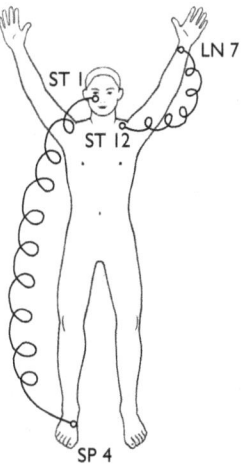

Figure 7-23 This example shows the two-cord sequence for treating the Lung Divergent Meridian.

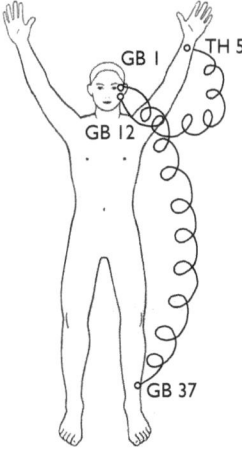

Figure 7-24 This example shows the two-cord sequence for treating the Gallbladder Divergent Meridian.

Treatment Summary

As earlier mentioned, one of Oriental medicine's main goals is to increase our patients' vitality and health by strengthening and supporting organ function. With a direct link to the organs, we would think that the Divergent Meridians would rank high among our treatment options. But largely because so little diagnostic and treatment information about this powerful system has been available, meridian-based therapists have had not had the opportunity to use it, limiting our ability to address more challenging situations.

Divergent Meridian treatments can have profound effects on an individual's overall health, but obviously only if the diagnosis and subsequent treatment are correct and thorough. The outcome will be evident in the balancing of all of the meridian systems. If we have been off base, there will be little apparent improvement in these.

In this chapter, we have discussed how jitsu Regular Meridian imbalances beyond the third degree are picked up by the Extra Meridians, while the Divergent Meridian system receives the kyo flow. Thus, we associate the Divergent Meridian system with the root or causes of an imbalance, while we associate the Extra Meridian system — and its jitsu-meridian connection — with the symptom side of an imbalance.

When we diagnose the Divergent Meridian system as being out of balance, we will always find the Extra Meridians out of balance too. With the advanced approaches available through Shin So Shiatsu, we can treat both systems at the same time. This is very similar to the "most kyo-most jitsu" Regular Meridian treatment (Chapter 5). I consider an imbalanced Divergent Meridian to be the "most kyo," and the imbalanced Extra Meridian to be the "most jitsu" of the whole ki-meridian system. My experience is that treating both the Divergent and the Extra meridians yields the best results.

Generally speaking, these deeper meridian treatments can be considered more honji in nature, since treating them creates stability in the whole energy matrix (i.e. when we rebalance the Divergent Meridians, the Extra and Regular meridian systems balance out). This is the purpose of a honji treatment, to re-establish balance in the whole energy system and thus create a foundation for illness prevention. However, because Extra and Divergent meridian treatments are also very effective at eliminating patient discomfort, I also consider them to be hyoji in nature. Therefore, these two systems can be considered the basis for both honji or hyoji treatments.

I generally follow a Divergent Meridian treatment with a Regular Meridian (in this case, hyoji) treatment. I have found it prudent to abbreviate this latter portion of a treatment to avoid over-stimulating the patient and triggering an uncomfortable reaction. Just how much of a Regular Meridian treatment you should give can only be determined on an individual basis.

8

Diagnosing and Treating
The Oceans System

spring tide —
piercing my entire body
the whistle from a boat

- Seishi Yamaguchi -

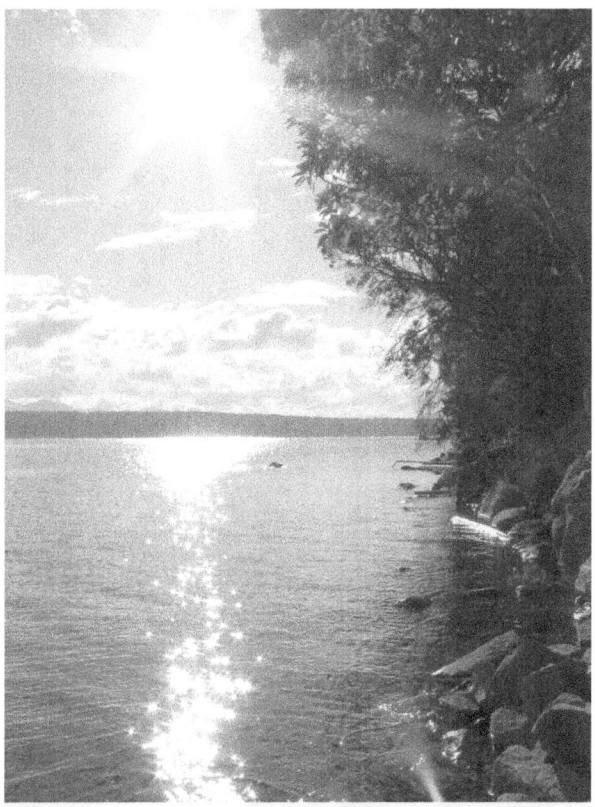

In this chapter, you will learn:

- How our grasp of the Regular Meridian system is essential to our work at this deeper energetic level.

- How to detect imbalance in the Oceans System.

- How to sense and diagnose the six Ocean zones.

- How to restore balance to the Oceans System via two simple methods.

Chapter 8

Diagnosing and Treating
The Oceans System

Our seemingly endless journey along the many energy rivers and tributaries of the body has carried us to the sweeping shores of a vast ocean. Before us lies the deepest, and probably the most mysterious, energy system within the human body.

The TCM View

TCM makes only sparse reference to the Oceans System. The classics identify Four Oceans — Sui-Koku Kai, the "Sea of Water and Grain;" Ki Kai, the "Sea of Qi;" Ketsu Kai, the "Sea of Blood;" and Zui Kai, the "Sea of Marrow" — and relates them to the four seas of Chinese mythology. These seas are linked to the continents by the 12 "great rivers," i.e. the meridians. We are told simply that when the body is out of balance, one of the Four Oceans will be either replete or deficient. For example, symptoms of imbalance in the Sea of Water and Grain include distension and fullness in the epigastric and abdominal areas, hunger with an inability to eat, and an inability to fully metabolize what has been ingested. If balance in the Oceans is not regained, death may follow.

Acupuncture points known to help regulate the Oceans are listed in figure 8-1, below.

Ocean	Regulating Points
Sui-Koku Kai Sea of Water and Grain	ST 36, ST 30
Ki Kai Sea of Qi	ST 9, GV 14, GV 15 CV 17, BL 10
Ketsu Kai Sea of Blood	ST 37, ST 39, BL 11
Zui Kai Sea of Marrow	GV 16, GV 17, GV 20

Figure 8-1 Oceans System Regulating Points as identified by TCM

Doctors Oda and Yoshimoto:
Oceans System Pioneers

The TCM view leaves us with many questions. What exactly is the function of the Oceans System in the human body? How is it linked to the Regular, Extra, and Divergent meridian systems? How can we diagnose whether or not the Oceans System needs treatment? Are there treatments that effectively regulate the Oceans?

At this threshold of my research, I found the pioneering work of two Japanese medical doctors, Hajime Oda and Hideo Yoshimoto, extremely helpful. Dr. Oda's research was invaluable in expanding my knowledge of the Oceans and provided me with the tools I needed to further explore this complex system. He had already developed a sound diagnostic system (figure 8-2) which I was able to adapt to my work with the Finger Test Method. He had also identified two Oceans in addition to the four cited by TCM: the Yin-Miyaku Kai (Yin Meridian Ocean) and Yo-Miyaku Kai (Yang Meridian Ocean). Dr. Yoshimoto, meanwhile, developed what he calls the Shi Kai (Four Oceans) method for diagnosing the Oceans System and found specific correspondences between patient symptoms and Ocean imbalances.

Oceans	Sound Images
Sui-Koku Kai	Loh
Yin-Miyaku Kai	Toh
Yo-Miyaku Kai	Te
Ketsu Kai	Su
Ki Kai	Na
Zui Kai	Ne

Figure 8-2 Sound images for the six Oceans developed by Dr. Hajime Oda.

Toward a More Complete Picture

Ki has universal dimensions. It not only flows within the human body, but is present with every expression of life throughout existence. All creation unfolds through the movement and exchange of ki.

Classical Chinese thought sees human beings as part of nature, a microcosm of the macrocosm, and it is only through the exchange of ki with the larger environment that we survive.

Within the human body, the Oceans represent the deepest energy system, the final destination for the 12 Regular and 8 Extra Meridians. But then, what happens? What do the Oceans do with all this ki? We might similarly ask why the Earth's land masses are not flooded by the seas.

The answer is evaporation. If the Oceans System is indeed the deepest energy reservoir within the human body, it is my contention that the only place for energy to flow from here is into the Cosmic System. The excess, or overflow, from our bodies dissipates into and influences the "small" Cosmic System around us.

This is what we have been calling ja ki (surface and internal) — the excess energy which disrupts communication between the energy matrix of the human body and the larger environment around us. As our meridian systems reach more serious levels of imbalance, greater quantities of ja ki accumulate and illnesses develop. Treating the Oceans helps eliminate this and re-establish a healthy energetic dialogue between the "small" and "large" Cosmic systems.

If we wish to effectively treat the Oceans System, it seems essential that we develop a more detailed geography of the meridians and Oceans. My own research suggests there are two main branches or "divides" of this meridian flow (shown in figure 8-3). One arises as the Regular Meridian system and flows into the Four Oceans. The other, it appears to me, is excess energy from the Extra Meridian system. It flows into the Yin-Miyaku Kai and Yo-Miyaku Kai, as identified by Dr. Oda. Overflow from very specific Regular and Extra meridians finds its way to specific Ocean zones. The energy which initially overflows from the Regular to the Extra Meridians never cycles back as such to the Regular Meridians, but ends up in the Oceans System, where it undergoes transformation.

Dr. Yoshimoto's research represents an important step in clarifying the relationships between specific meridians and Oceans. He cites the following correlations between patient symptoms and imbalances in the Shi Kai (Four Oceans):

1. **Sui-Koku Kai:** almost all digestive disorders, including digestive tract cancers. The stomach, large intestine, liver, and pancreas are often involved.

2. **Ketsu Kai:** disorders involving the genital organs and endocrine system; includes cancer of the female organs.

3. **Ki Kai:** lung disorders; includes lung and breast cancer.

4. **Zui Kai:** dysfunction of the brain and entire nervous system.

Dr. Yoshimoto has found that conventional energy treatments yield negligible results once imbalances have reached the stage where such serious illnesses as cancer are present. He concludes, however, that without knowledge of the Shi Kai systems and the application of concomitant treatments, there is almost no possibility of improving these conditions.

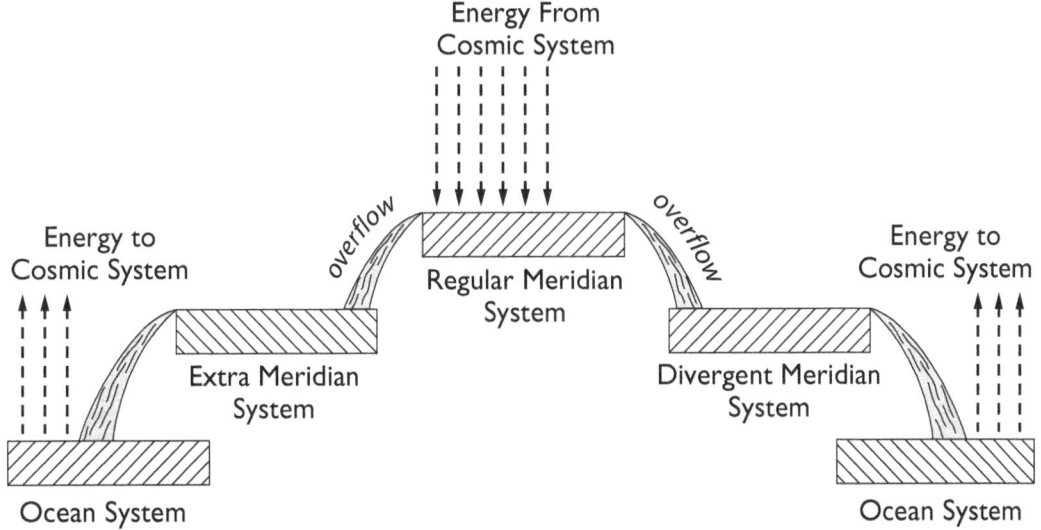

Figure 8-3 Two branches of energy flow into the Oceans.

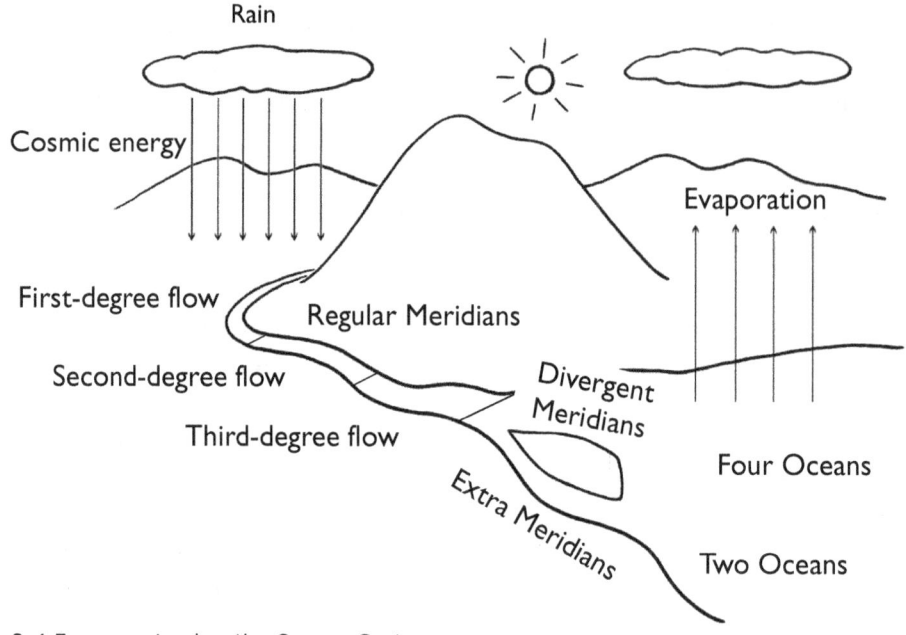

Figure 8-4 From sea to sky: the Oceans System

The Saito Ocean Zones

The Oceans System appears to receive energy flow primarily from the Regular and Extra meridian systems. The Four Oceans (Shi Kai) absorb Regular Meridian flow; the Yin- and Yo-Miyaku Kai absorb Extra Meridian flow. Using the Oceans sensor (figure 8-10) and sound images (figure 8-2), I have been able to sense and map six Ocean zones as they appear on the abdomen (figure 8-9).

One of my primary research goals was to clarify the relationships between the Regular and Extra meridians and the Oceans zones. There are six Oceans zones ostensibly receiving flow from 12 Regular and 8 Extra meridians — 20 meridians in all. But which meridians flow where? The answer came as something as a surprise to me: each of the six Oceans receives overflow from just one meridian. This is illustrated in figures 8-5 and 8-6.

Four Oceans	Regular Meridian
1. Sui-Koku Kai	Stomach Regular Meridian energy
2. Ketsu Kai	Liver Regular Meridian energy
3. Ki Kai	Spleen Regular Meridian energy
4. Zui Kai	Kidney Regular Meridian energy

Figure 8-5 Regular Meridian flow into the Oceans

Two Oceans	Extra Meridian
1. Yin-Miyaku Kai	Penetrating Meridian (Triple Heater Meridian)
2. Yo-Miyaku Kai	Belt Meridian (Heart Constrictor Meridian)

Figure 8-6 Extra Meridian flow into the Oceans

Where They Flow:
The Ocean Meridians

In our earlier exploration of the Extra Meridians (Chapter 6), we learned that all of the yin Regular Meridians overflow into the yang Extra Meridians, while all of the yang Regular Meridians overflow into the yin Extra Meridians. Now, looking at figures 8-5 and 8-6, we see that only four Regular Meridians — Stomach, Spleen, Liver, and Kidney — flow into the Ocean zones. Why only four? What of the other Regular Meridians?

The same phenomenon occurs with the Extra Meridians — only two flow into the Ocean zones. What happens to the remaining six?

Meridian Fundamentals

My conclusion is that these four Regular Meridians—the Stomach, Spleen, Liver and Kidney—play the most vital roles in the human body. The Spleen Meridian is essential in creating and maintaining our supply of ki; the Liver Meridian is profoundly involved in the storage and maintenance of Blood; the Kidney Meridian manages body Fluids. The Stomach Meridian, known as the "King of the Regular Meridians," governs them all—without the Stomach we will have neither ki, nor Blood, nor Fluids. Yet when we have an optimal balance of all of these substances, then we have optimal health.

If, for some reason, energy overflow from one of these four Regular Meridians reaches the Oceans System, and we treat it, we are in effect balancing the entire Regular Meridian system. The remaining eight meridians are of course very important to our overall health. But, returning to our metaphor of waterways in nature, we can see how these latter eight meridians behave like tributaries, while the first four comprise the main stream. When the main stream is flowing smoothly, we don't need to worry about tributary flow.

Note that in Chapter 5 we discussed the importance of a slightly different list of four Regular Meridians: the Liver, Kidney, Stomach, and Large Intestine. In that context, we were observing how those four meridians work together to create and distribute ki. For optimum function within the ki meridian system, we need a balance in the function of these four meridians.

The four meridians we are discussing with regard to the Oceans (Stomach, Spleen, Kidney, Liver) have an impact outside of the ki meridian system alone — they govern the whole body via its essential substances.

When we find imbalances in the Oceans, we are considering a quite different scenario than imbalances within the Regular Meridians alone. When the Oceans become affected, this means that imbalance in the meridian system has been significant or has persisted for some time, and at a very deep level. When this happens, organ function is compromised, and our body's ability to create and circulate essential substances (including but not limited to ki) is impaired. This can lead to serious consequences for our physical organism, and reflects the gravity of a persistent Oceans-level imbalance.

In terms of the Extra Meridians, we find a similar situation: the Belt and Penetrating meridians regulate the whole Extra Meridian system. There is much still to know about the Extra Meridians, yet we can speculate as follows. First, we know that the Heart Constrictor Meridian flows into the Belt Meridian, while the Triple Heater Meridian flows into the Penetrating Meridian. We might be able to appreciate their importance just by virtue of their respective locations, at the centre of the yin and yang side of each arm and leg. Figure 8-7 presents an interesting view of this meridian to body-structure relationship.

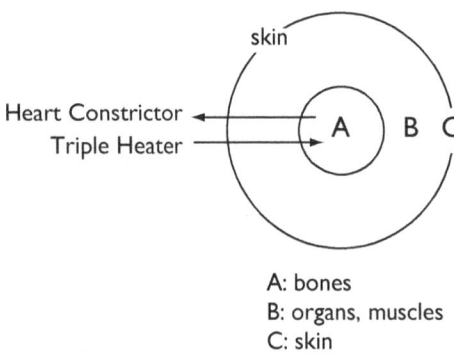

Figure 8-7 Meridians, their functions, and body structure

Section A: Bones, Brain, and Heart

Section A here represents the skeletal system (bones), centrally located so as to support the body structurally. Meridian functions associated with section A are those of the Kidney and Bladder. This same meridian pair also maintains functions of the brain and nervous system, and the endocrine system, and altogether these can be said to control the functioning of the whole human body.

Two more very important meridians associated with section A are the Heart and Small Intestine. Humans are said to be "emotional animals" and the maintenance of our complex emotional system falls to this meridian pair. The Heart Meridian engages both emotional as well as heart organ functions. So, in section A, we have essentially, the brain and heart functions, neither of which we can live without.

Section B: Muscles and Organs

Between the bones and the skin is space for the muscles and the organs. The meridians most engaged with the muscular system are the Liver and Gallbladder.

Section B is also the domain of the Stomach and Spleen meridians. As we already appreciate, the Stomach Meridian plays a role in governing all of the Regular Meridians.

Section C: Skin

Skin functions are regulated by the Lung and Large Intestine meridians. The responsibilities borne by this meridian pair are far from superficial however. Their role is not simply to exchange waste products for fresh ones, but to regulate and transport Cosmic energy throughout the meridian system, located just beneath the skin. The Lung and Large Intestine are central in the release of ja ki through the meridians to the skin and in the reception of fresh Cosmic energy into the meridian system.

The Heart Constrictor and Triple Heater meridians are associated with sections C and A. One of the Heart Constrictor's primary functions is blood circulation. This process begins with the Heart (section A), which sees blood pumped outward (toward section C) and then returned (to A). The Heart Constrictor also circulates "emotional current" from the outside (section C) to section A(the Heart Meridian) and back again.

The Triple Heater Divergent Meridian connects all the organs by transmitting information from section A to section C in order to maintain optimal functioning and health. It also protects the body from intruders; and in keeping with this, sends certain signals to our control centre in section A.

Our diagnosis of the Oceans System makes much more sense when we fully grasp Regular Meridian functions and actually learn to read what is happening inside the patient's body.

The Ocean Meridians

In the course of my research, I realized that each Ocean zone has its own Ocean Meridian. For example, figure 8-8 shows the Ki Kai (Sea of Qi) zone on the abdomen transected by a meridian, which on the arm and leg overlaps with the Regular Spleen Meridian in first-degree. This suggests a relationship between the Ki Kai Ocean zone and the Spleen Regular Meridian. Meridians similarly transect each of the remaining five Ocean zones on the abdomen, overlapping pathways corresponding to the Stomach, Liver, Kidney, Triple Heater, and Heart Constrictor Regular meridians in first degree.

I see this as the process by which fresh Cosmic energy destined for the Ocean zones enters the meridians via the fingertips and toes, and excess energy is discharged via the same route.

It is important to note that when these Ocean meridians are in a state of balance, they are not detectable with the finger test. Only two conditions render an Ocean meridian detectable by the finger test:

1. When energetic imbalance has reached the Oceans level: i.e. the overflow energy from a Regular or Extra meridian is being accepted by an Ocean, and this Ocean meridian is exerting itself to contain the imbalance. This would coincide with a positive (sticky) test result using the "Na" sound and testing over the abdomen with our open palm (see below).

2. When "residual accumulation" of overflow reaches a certain level within an Ocean Meridian. In this case, an Ocean has accepted overflow energy (perhaps on a number of occasions) without necessarily going out of balance. At the present moment, the patient may only present with an imbalance in the Extra or Divergent systems; yet this Ocean Meridian is trying to release its accumulated energy to the Cosmic System for transformation. We can imagine this accumulation of energy to be like the gradual build up of sediment on the ocean floor. In these cases, we may be able to sense the beginnings of an Oceans System imbalance in the Ocean Meridians of the arms and legs. Even before it is apparent in the Ocean zones of the hara, we can detect this, and begin to treat it.

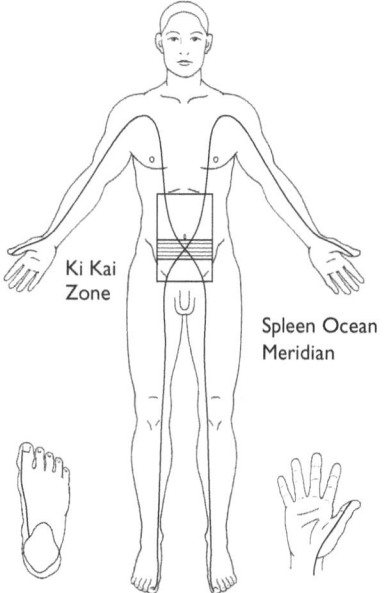

Figure 8-8 The Ki Kai zone and Spleen Ocean Meridian

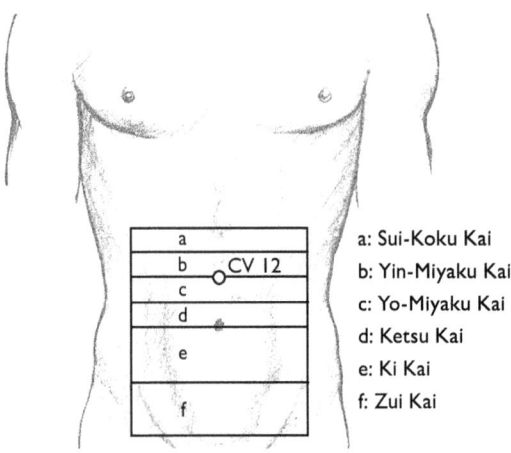

Figure 8-9 Saito Ocean zones on the abdomen

a: Sui-Koku Kai
b: Yin-Miyaku Kai
c: Yo-Miyaku Kai
d: Ketsu Kai
e: Ki Kai
f: Zui Kai

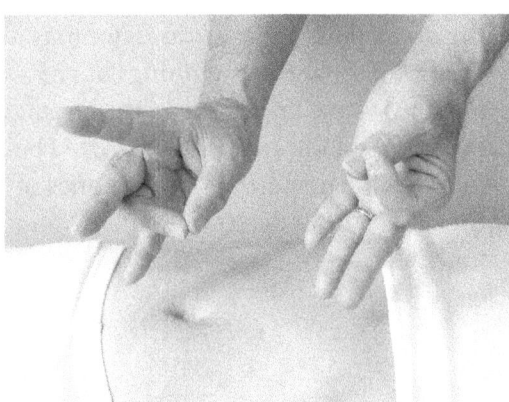

Figure 8-10 Oceans sensor

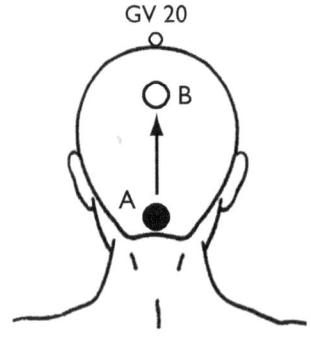

Figure 8-11 Oceans System confirmation point

Instruction
Diagnosing imbalances in the Oceans System

1. To determine whether the Oceans System is out of balance, place the palm of your hand over your patient's tanden and image the sound "Na." If the finger test elicits a sticky response, the answer is yes.

2. Use the Saito Oceans Diagnostic Chart (figure 8-9) to determine which Oceans zone requires treatment. Place your general sensor over each of the six Ocean zones in sequence from "a" to "f" and image the sound associated with each one. When the finger test elicits a sticky response you have found the out-of-balance zone. You can also use your Oceans sensor (figure 8-10) over each of the Ocean zones and image the question, "which zone is vibrating."

3. To confirm this Oceans System imbalance, check the regulating point along the centre line at the back of the head (figure 8-11). Image the sound "Na." When the Oceans System is in balance, finger testing this point at position A using the Oceans System sensor will always elicit a sticky response. When the Oceans System is out of balance, the point travels upwards along the centre line of the head and toward GV 20. The point at position A will no longer feel sticky; you will obtain this response at position B instead.

Treating the Oceans System

I have found ja ki removal to be the most effective technique for restoring balance to the deeper energy systems. Two approaches are described below: Method 2, using the Mu Bun Sai Chart, is somewhat simpler and usually takes less time to complete.

Instruction — Method 1
Treating the Oceans System with two-point ja ki removal

1. Once you have diagnosed which Ocean zone is out of balance, position the patient for treatment as follows (figure 8-12 to 8-14). Gently grasp the patient's ankle with your hand in the Oceans sensor position. Select the appropriate sound image for the Ocean zone requiring treatment. For example, if you have diagnosed imbalance in the Ki Kai zone, image the sound "Na," and gently slide the patient's leg downward. As the heel of one leg reaches the mid-calf area of the second leg, the finger test will register sticky.

2. Once the leg is in position, place your Oceans sensor over the Ki Kai diagnostic zone on the hara. If the leg position is correct, this zone will no longer be vibrating: i.e. the finger test will now be smooth.

3. Next, position the arm (in this case, the arm on the opposite side of the leg you have just positioned.) Grasp the patient's wrist, image the sound "Na," and slowly slide the arm down, within the Oceans zone, as shown in figure 8-14. When the arm is correctly

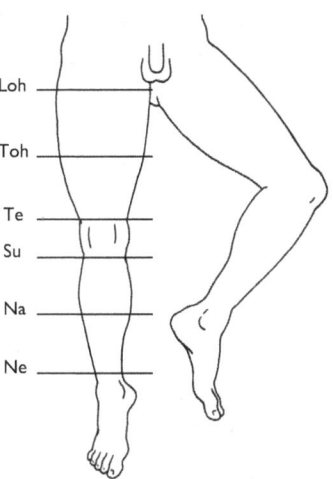

Figure 8-12 Oceans treatment leg positions

Sound Images	Oceans	Associated Meridians
Loh	Sui-Koku Kai	Stomach
Toh	Yin-Miyaku Kai	Triple Heater
Te	Yo-Miyaku Kai	Heart Constrictor
Su	Ketsu Kai	Liver
Na	Ki Kai	Spleen
Ne	Zui Kai	Kidney

Figure 8-13 Oceans zones in the leg

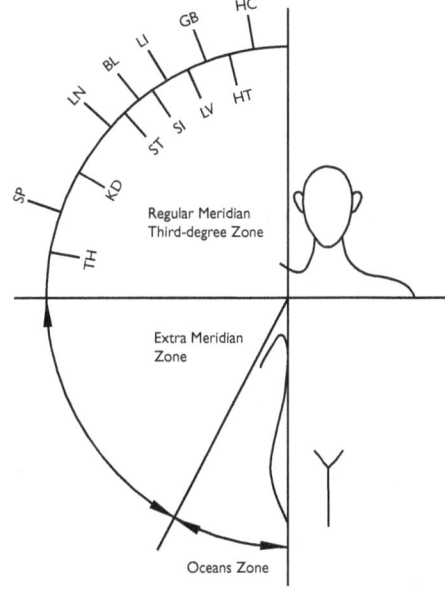

Figure 8-14 Arm positions for Oceans treatment

placed, the finger test will register sticky over the Ki Kai zone.

4. The Ki Kai zone receives Spleen Meridian overflow: once the arm and leg have been correctly positioned, first-degree flow for the Spleen Meridian will be activated on the arm and leg.

5. Place your point sensor on the Spleen Meridian activated in this bending position, image the question, where is the "Shin So Ja ki Point," and trace your sensor along the meridian line on the lower leg until you sense one sticky point.

6. Follow the same procedure for the lower arm.

7. Place the middle fingers of each hand gently on these sticky points, hold them, and observe the release of ja ki from the patient's body.

8. Treat the second arm and leg in the same way.

9. Proceed with a whole body shiatsu treatment.

Instruction — Method 2
Treating the Oceans System with Mu Bun Sai ja ki removal

Refer to your Mu Bun Sai Ja Ki Chart (figure 6-29a,b and *Reference Manual*).

1. Follow steps 1-4 in Method 1, above.

2. Once the patient's leg and arm have been positioned, gently place your palm on the Spleen zone as shown on the Mu Bun Sai chart. Follow the complete ja ki removal procedure as you have done for the Extra and Divergent meridian systems. Remember to treat both sides of the body and follow with a general shiatsu treatment.

Although there may be no indication our Ocean zones are out of balance, it is wise to check the Ocean Meridians. If we do detect an early accumulation of "sediment" there, we can increase our potential for sustained health and our overall vitality by following the Oceans treatments outlined above.

Instruction
Detecting early imbalances in the Ocean Meridians

1. Using your general sensor and Oceans sound images, finger test the first-degree Regular Meridian locations for the legs or arms.

2. If you get a sticky response, for example, when you image the sound "Loh" over the Stomach Meridian on the leg, then Sui-Koku Kai (Sea of Water and Grain) would benefit from treatment.

3. Follow one of the two treatment procedures outlined above.

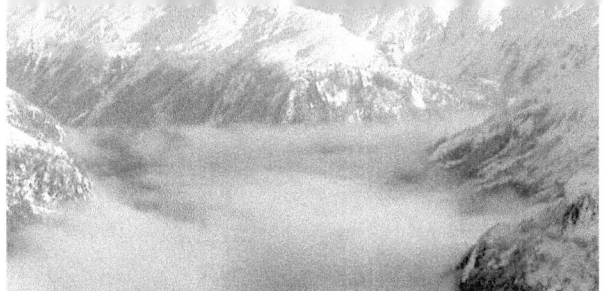

9

Diagnosing and Treating
The Tai Kyoku System

from the cage
fireflies one by one
turn into stars

- Seisensui Ogiwara -

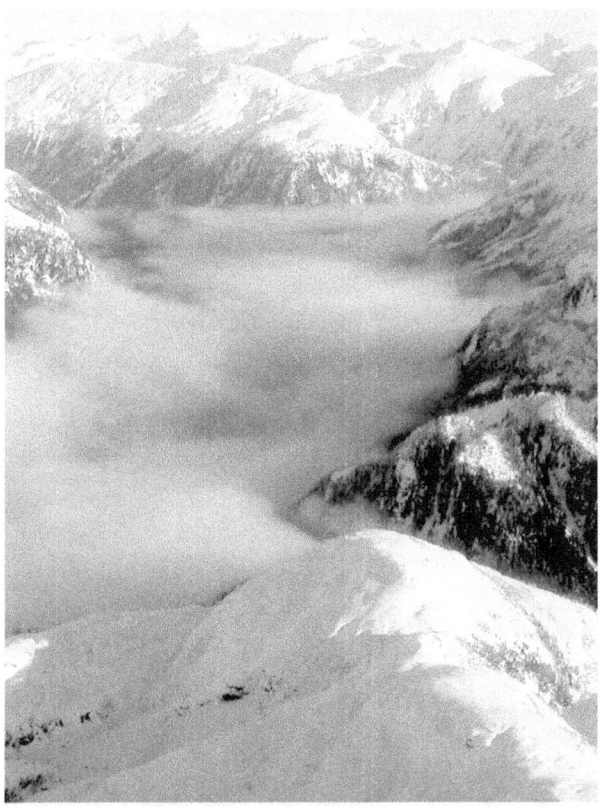

In this chapter, you will learn:

- How to sense the Tai Kyoku System's unusual spiral meridians.

- How to diagnose a Tai Kyoku imbalance and confirm that diagnosis.

- How to treat the Tai Kyoku System by removing ja ki.

Chapter 9

Diagnosing and Treating
The Tai Kyoku System

Cosmic energy is engaged in a constant interplay with our body's energetic matrix. As long as we are alive, and whether we are healthy or not, we receive energy from the cosmos and release it back again via our meridian complex. It is only at the point of death — or the final separation of our yin and yang energies — that this exchange ceases.

Shin So Shiatsu sees two distinctive components in this interplay. The first, little known or studied, is what I have called the Tai Kyoku System. In Japanese, it means simply the "cosmic" or "universal" energy system. The second component is the Chakra System, familiar to many who have explored certain yoga and meditation techniques. It is covered briefly as Chapter 10.

When a state of "dis-ease" surpasses the point where the ki meridian system can bring it into check, the Tai Kyoku System becomes engaged in a further, and sometimes final attempt to support the body. If we are unable to regain balance via this system, we may not expect healing to occur through a meridian-energetic approach. We rarely encounter this level of imbalance in our clinical practices. When a patient's Tai Kyoku meridians do reflect the occasional upset, I don't get overly concerned. The individual may be experiencing a period of particularly high stress — physically, mentally, or emotionally — that has temporarily created such an energy imbalance. These states are generally short lived and easily resolved.

When the Tai Kyoku System is more chronically engaged, however, a more serious health problem is indicated.

Where they Flow:
Tai Kyoku Meridians

Tai Kyoku meridians flow in an unusual pattern. Unlike the vertical and horizontal pathways traversed by the body's other energy systems, they follow a spiral pattern as shown in figures 9-1 and 9-2.

When Tai Kyoku 1 (yang) and 2 (yin) are called upon to deal with an energetic imbalance, large energy circles appear on the abdominal and back areas (figures 9-3 and 9-4). These are "energetic exchange zones" through which energy is transferred from the outside in and the inside out.

Figure 9-5 shows the flow of Tai Kyoku 1 energy through the entire body. This meridian system receives only yang energy (Large Intestine, Triple Heater, Small Intestine, Stomach, Gallbladder, and Bladder) which enters the body via the fingertips and exits via the toes. While this Tai Kyoku 1 chart shows the meridian as a single pathway, it actually consists of six parallel energy lines (figure 9-6) that ultimately meet at the ankle and wrist.

Figure 9-7 shows the flow of Tai Kyoku 2 energy throughout the body. This meridian system receives only yin energy which flows into the body at the ends of the toes, travels up to the fingertips, and then out of the body. While this chart shows Tai Kyoku 2 as a single pathway, it carries six yin meridians (Lung, Heart Constrictor, Heart, Spleen, Liver, and Kidney) running parallel to one another (figure 9-8). These six meridians meet at a very particular point just below the inner ankle and wrist.

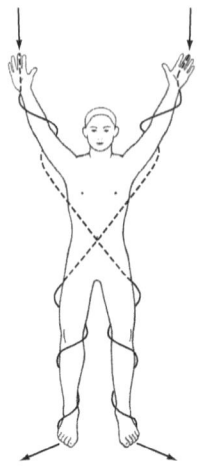

Figure 9-1 The spiral flow characterizing the Tai Kyoku 1 (yang) meridians. We can see how this cosmic energy enters and exits our bodies through the tips of our fingers and toes.

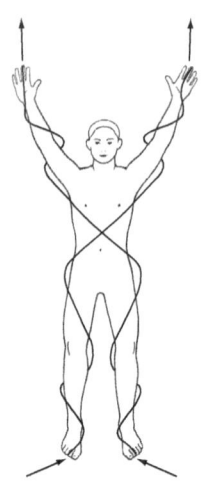

Figure 9-2 The spiral energy flow characterizing the Tai Kyoku 2 (yin) meridians.

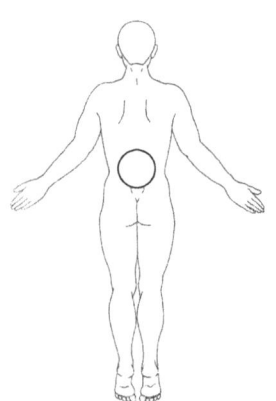

Figure 9-3 When Tai Kyoku 1 is activated, an energy circle appears on the back.

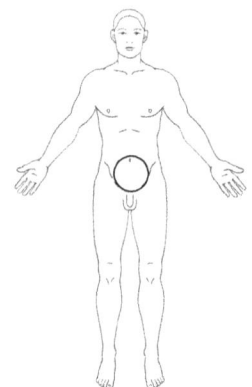

Figure 9-4 When Tai Kyoku 2 is activated, an energy circle will appear on the abdomen.

143 SHIN SO SHIATSU

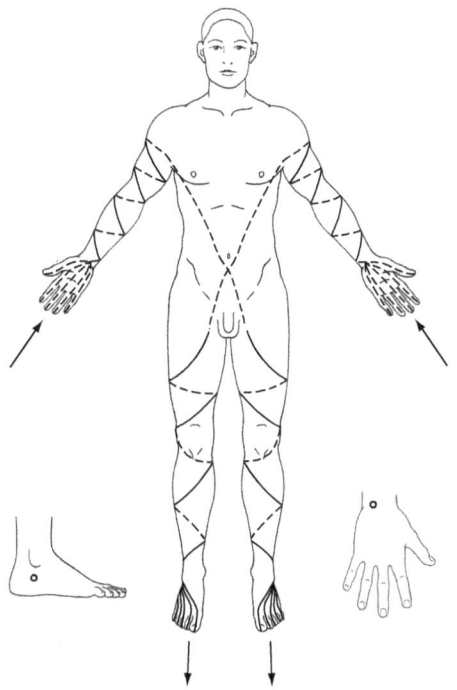

Figure 9-5 Tai Kyoku 1 as it flows throughout the body and treatment points on the wrist and ankle

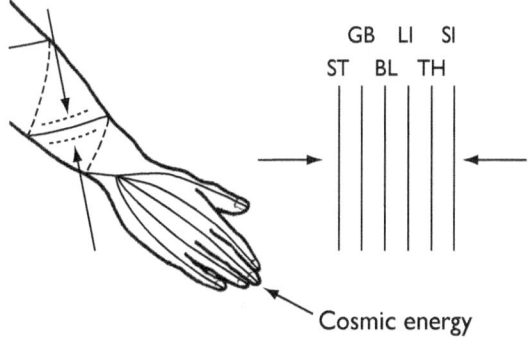

Figure 9-6 Tai Kyoku 1 consists of six yang energy pathways.

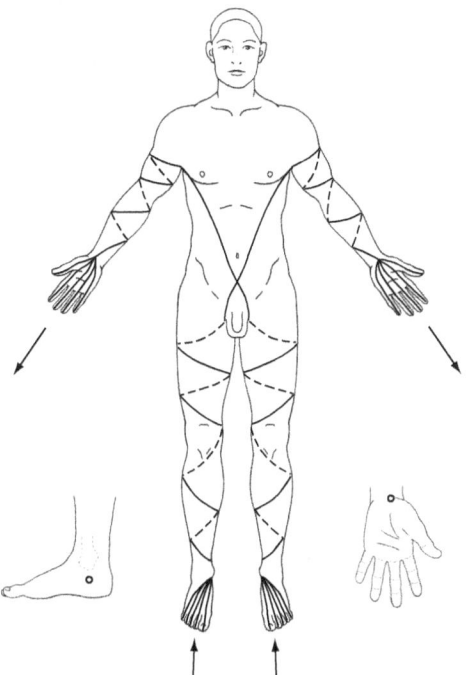

Figure 9-7 Tai Kyoku 2 as it flows throughout the body and treatment points on the wrist and ankle

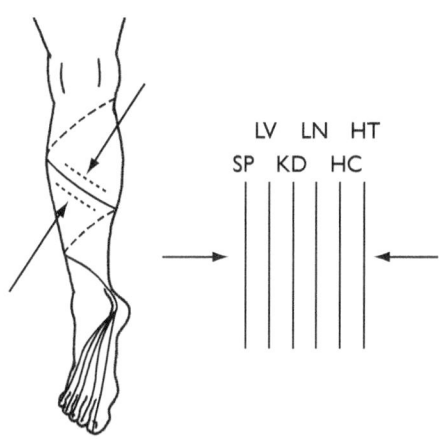

Figure 9-8 Tai Kyoku 2 consists of six yin energy pathways.

Diagnosing the Tai Kyoku System

In a Tai Kyoku imbalance, as with the meridian systems we have already explored, we are able to sense which organ/meridian system is involved. We can therefore discern which Regular Meridian most needs our attention.

Instruction
Diagnosing Tai Kyoku 1

1. Place your Tai Kyoku 1 sensor (figure 9-9) over the patient's tanden and image the sound "Gu." If the finger test elicits a sticky sensation, the Tai Kyoku 1 system is out of balance.

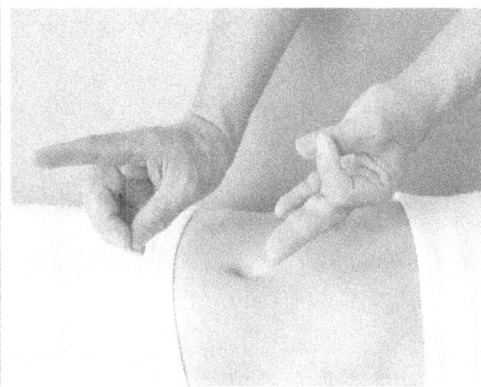

Figure 9-9 Tai Kyoku 1 sensor

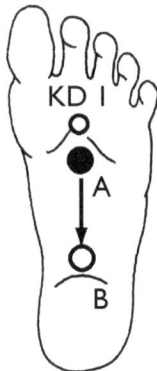

Figure 9-10 Tai Kyoku 1 confirmation point

2. Confirmation points for Tai Kyoku 1 are on the bottom of the foot (figure 9-10). Use your Tai Kyoku 1 sensor and finger test. When this system is in balance, you will get a sticky response at point A. When the system is out of balance, you will get a smooth response at point A and a sticky response somewhere between points A and B.

3. When the Tai Kyoku 1 system is out of balance, one meridian will elicit a sticky response. To diagnose which Tai Kyoku 1 meridian is out of balance, place your Tai Kyoku 1 sensor on the patient's lower arm as indicated by the arrow in figure 9-6. Image the name of each yang Regular Meridian and finger test.

Instruction
Diagnosing Tai Kyoku 2

1. Place your Tai Kyoku 2 sensor (figure 9-11) over the tanden, image the sound "Ka," and finger test. A sticky response tells you this system requires treatment.

2. Confirmation points for Tai Kyoku 2 are on the palm of the hand (figure 9-12). Use your Tai Kyoku 2 sensor and finger test. When this system is in balance, you will get a sticky response at point A. When the system is out of balance, you will get a smooth response at point A. You will detect stickiness, or imbalance, somewhere between points A and B.

3. To ascertain which of the Tai Kyoku 2 meridians is creating this imbalance,

we follow the same approach as for the Tai Kyoku 1 system, substituting the Tai Kyoku 2 sensor and imaging the names of the six yin Regular Meridians (figure 9-8).

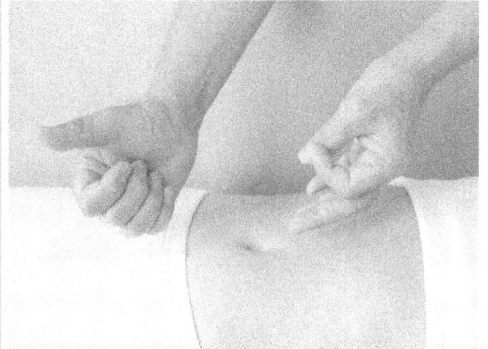

Figure 9-11 Tai Kyoku 2 sensor

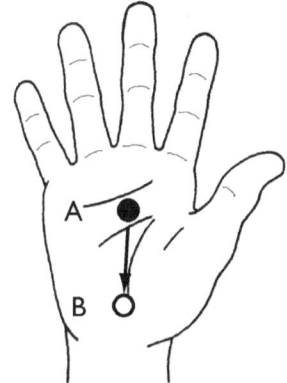

Figure 9-12 Tai Kyoku 2 confirmation point

Treating the Tai Kyoku System

I have found ja ki removal to be the most effective way of restoring balance to this deeper energy system.

Instruction

Treating the Tai Kyoku system by removing ja ki

When treating the Tai Kyoku System, it is not necessary to set the patient's arms and legs in particular positions as we have with preceding systems. Ask them to lie comfortably, face up.

1. Place the middle fingers of your left and right hands at each of two points on opposite sides of the patient's body, one on the wrist and one just below the ankle. If you have diagnosed a Tai Kyoku 1 imbalance, refer to figure 9-5. For Tai Kyoku 2, see figure 9-7.

2. Hold the points for approximately 30 seconds until you sense internal ja ki rising from the surface of the body. Release the points and wait until you sense via the finger test, that this ja ki has completely cleared. Treat the opposite side of the body.

3. Position your patient face down and follow with ja ki removal along the back (see Chapter 6, "Treating the Extra Meridians by removing ja ki").

4. Finish with a gentle shiatsu treatment to the whole body.

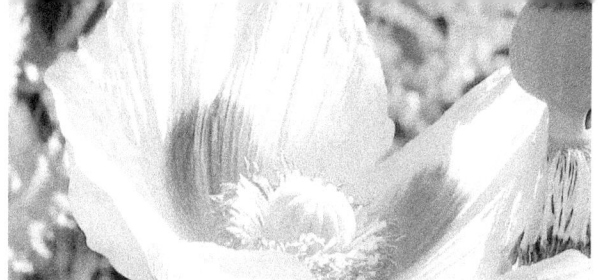

10

Diagnosing and Treating
The Chakra System

with plum blossom scent
this sudden sun emerges
along a mountain trail

- Basho -

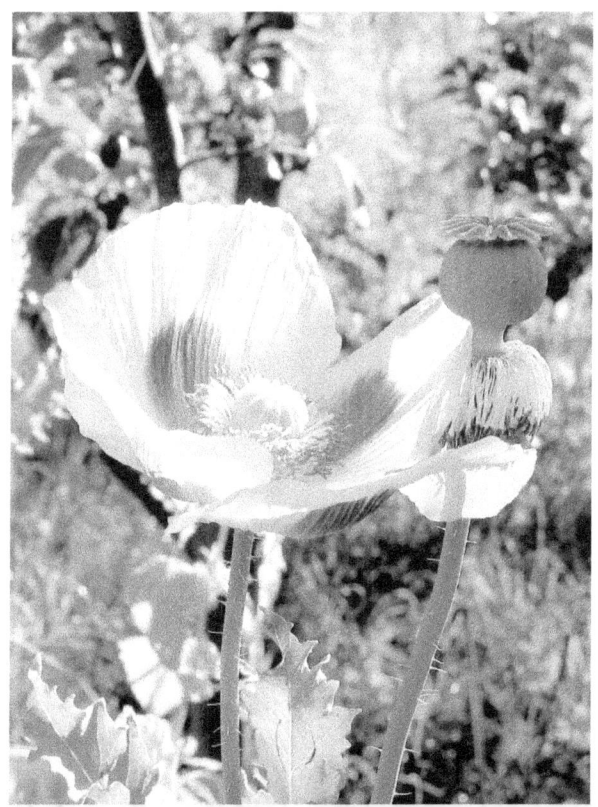

In this chapter, you will learn:

- How to sense which chakras are open and which are closed.

- How to sense the Chakra Meridian.

- How to open chakras.

Chapter 10

Diagnosing and Treating
The Chakra System

Although not formally discussed in the fields of shiatsu and acupuncture, the chakras strongly influence our health on physical, mental, and emotional levels. Other healing approaches do focus on this component of our energy matrix. I strongly recommend Barbara Ann Brennan's thorough and insightful book, *Hands of Light: A Guide to Healing Through the Human Energy Field* (Bantam Books, New York, 1987).

In this chapter, I will simply explain how to integrate chakras into the Shin So Shiatsu system in order to fully optimize the healing effects of our work.

Our sensor for the Chakra System (figure 10-1) was first identified by Dr. Hideo Yoshimoto. Using it in conjunction with the finger test, we can sense the locations of the seven major and twenty-one minor chakras (figure 10-2).

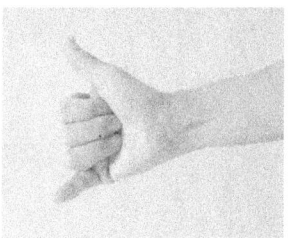

Figure 10-1 Yoshimoto Chakra sensor

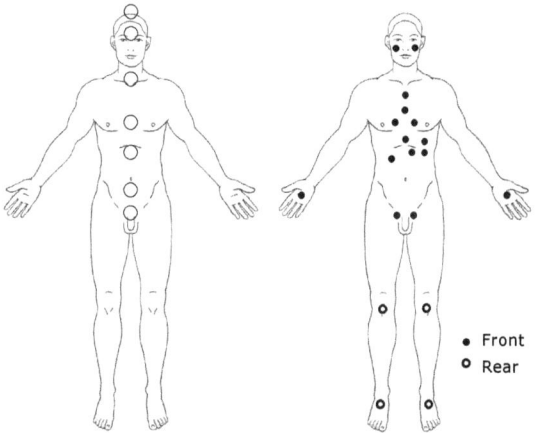

● Front
○ Rear

Figure 10-2 The seven major and twenty-one minor chakras (two lie behind the eyes).

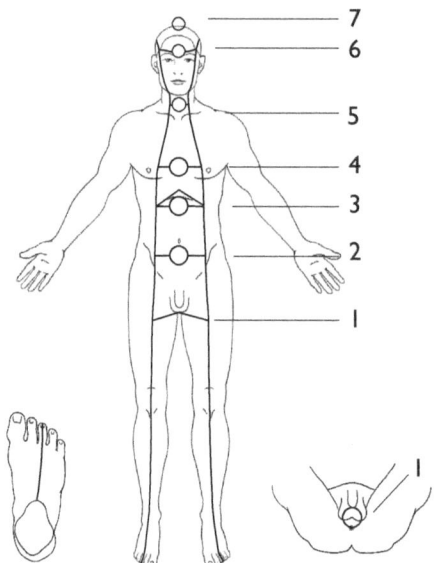

Figure 10-3 Chakra Meridian links the seven major chakras.

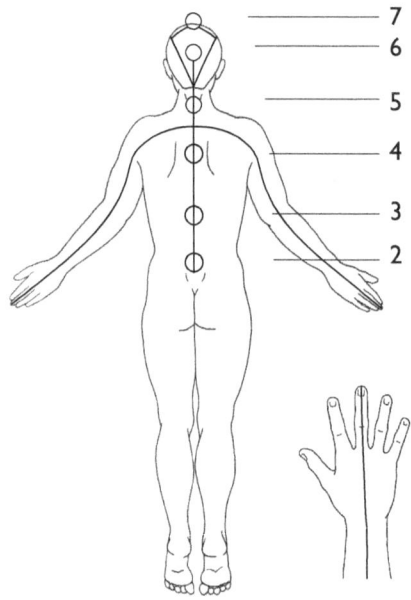

Figure 10-4 Chakra Meridian on back

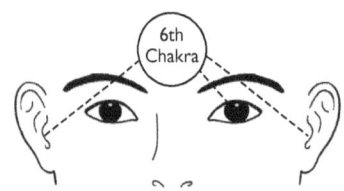

Figure 10-6 The 6th Chakra

Toward a More Complete Picture

My own research has led me to the discovery of the Chakra Meridian (figures 10-3 and 10-4) which links the seven major chakras. It is my belief that this Chakra Meridian system is independent of the meridian systems we have explored so far.

Using the chakra sensor, we are able to sense the energetic links between the chakras and certain organs and parts of the body (figure 10-5). Figure 10-6, for example, illustrates how the 6th Chakra governs the functions of the ears and left eye via an extended pathway (shown as broken lines).

	Chakra	Associated endocrine gland and areas governed by chakra
1	Base	adrenals: spinal column, kidneys
2	Sacral	gonads: reproductive system
3	Solar plexus	pancreas: stomach, liver, gallbladder, nervous system
4	Heart	thymus: circulatory system, heart, blood, vagus nerve
5	Throat	thyroid: lungs, alimentary canal, vocal and bronchial functions
6	Head	pituitary: lower brain, nervous system, ears, nose, left eye
7	Crown	pineal: upper brain, right eye

Figure 10-5 Chakras and their links with the organs

Instruction
Diagnosing chakras

For optimum health, it is important that our major and minor chakras are open, in other words, receiving fresh Cosmic energy. To determine whether a particular chakra is open:

1. Place your chakra sensor three to four inches above each chakra (make sure the "palm side" of your sensor is facing the chakra) and finger test. Open chakras will elicit a sticky response.

2. Sense the Chakra Meridian. Place your chakra sensor thumb side down on the surface of the body where the chakra meridian is located (figures 10-3 and 10-4). Gently slide your sensor across the meridian and finger test. When your chakra sensor crosses the Chakra Meridian the finger test will register sticky, unless the meridian is not vibrating. In this latter case, use the chakra sound image "oo." You will then be able to sense the location of the Chakra Meridian.

3. Sense the minor chakras. Position your chakra sensor with the little finger facing downward and finger test (figure 10-2). A sticky response tells you a minor chakra is open; a smooth response tells you it is closed.

Instruction
Treating the chakras using IP cords

Closed chakras elicit a smooth response with the finger test.

1. Determine which chakras are closed.

2. If, for example, the second chakra is closed, attach your IP cord to points (a) and (b) as shown in figure 10-7.

3. If you have diagnosed that chakras 2, 4, and 5 are closed, treat the lowest chakra, or in this case, the second chakra, and all the higher chakras will also open.

4. To determine which clip (red or black) should be attached to which point (a or b), touch the clips to each point respectively and finger test. Attach the clip to the point that elicits a smooth response.

5. To confirm you have attached the clips to the correct points, use your ja ki sensor and sense for ja ki releasing all over the body.

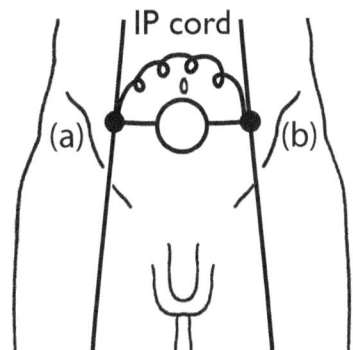

Figure 10-7 Treating Chakras

In Conclusion

Epilogue

Celebrating Milestones

It seems this year is a special milestone in my life as a shiatsu therapist.

It is the 40th year since I decided to study shiatsu and entered shiatsu school. It is also the 35th year since I moved to Canada and introduced Canadians to shiatsu for the first time.

It is also a milestone in that Shizuto Masunaga passed away 25 years ago.

I am glad to be publishing my book, *Shin So Shiatsu – Healing the Deeper Meridian Systems*, in this particular year of my life. I would like to express my deep gratitude to all of my shiatsu colleagues who have contributed their time and energy to this undertaking.

I feel so fortunate to have had such dedicated teachers and colleagues in the past 40 years of my professional life. Without their help, I never would have accomplished my work in the field of shiatsu.

In 1971, when I moved to North America, no one was practicing shiatsu therapy. I still remember the first 10 years and the challenges I faced in promoting shiatsu and keeping the business going. It was not rare for me to be working seven days a week during this period.

After Masunaga Sensei passed away in 1981, I became heavily involved in research and developing the Shin So Shiatsu approach. My shiatsu life became even more challenging.

I treated patients six days a week from morning until evening, taught students several days of the week, and in the late evenings after I got home, continued with my studies and the compilation of my research until after midnight. This lasted for more than 15 years.

When I think back, I wonder how I could have done so much work. The answer is that I was much younger, fueled by a lot of energy and great passion for my work.

But I realize how much of my private life with my family I sacrificed to this intensity of work. I truly appreciate all the support and understanding my family gave me. Without their help, it would have been impossible for me to accomplish what I did.

Undoubtedly, meridian shiatsu has become the main shiatsu approach in North America and Europe. But I wonder, myself, how much progress there has been in meridian shiatsu theory, diagnosis, and practice since Masunaga died 25 years ago.

We practitioners must cooperate with each other in order to create a more powerful meridian shiatsu approach and push beyond the level established by Masunaga. It will be my great pleasure if this book contributes to this. I am so sure our Masunaga Sensei is waiting for this day to come.

Finally, I would like to thank the members of Shin So Shiatsu International who have contributed their time and energy to helping me publish this book. I am especially proud of the members of Shin So Shiatsu British Columbia who have undertaken the editing, design, illustrations, layout, and even the photography. Special thanks to Cheryl Coull, for without her hard work this book never would have been published.

About Tetsuro Saito

The Father of Shiatsu in Canada

Tetsuro (Ted) Saito is one of the world's few shiatsu masters – one of only a handful of practitioners who has spent a lifetime fully dedicated to developing shiatsu and its healing potential.

He was born in the small Japanese city of Noda in 1941, just four months before the outbreak of World War Two. As a small child, he found joy in playing along the banks of the Edo River, and grew up with a deep love for nature and people. In university, he nurtured a passion for mountaineering, excelled in sciences, and became an electrical engineer. Soon however, he was drawn to another field, one with ancient roots and seemingly endless possibilities. Oriental medicine was experiencing a rebirth in Japan, particularly in the area of shiatsu. Saito entered the Japan Shiatsu School under masters Tokujiro Namikoshi and Shizuto Masunaga in 1966 and graduated in 1968.

In 1971, he travelled to North America and chose Toronto as the base for his new life. He established the Shiatsu Centre, treated patients who came in such numbers they were lined up at the door, trained students to become therapists, and invited others from Japan who would eventually open their own shiatsu centres and schools in Canada.

Saito is affectionately known as the "father of shiatsu in Canada," but his influence on shiatsu and energy work has rippled worldwide. He is founding director of Shin So Shiatsu International and supports hundreds of dedicated post-graduate students in North America, Europe, and Australia. He continues to research, maintains a busy shiatsu practice in Toronto, and lives with his wife Kathi in nearby Scarborough, not far from their daughters, Monika and Olivia.

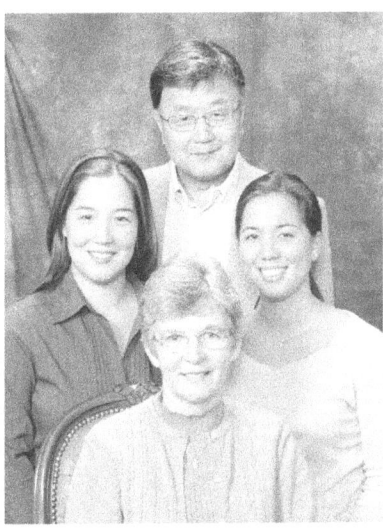

Shin So Shiatsu Studies

Shin So Shiatsu workshops are taught in North America, Europe, and Australia.

General Inquiries:
Shin So Shiatsu International
www.shinso-shiatsu.com

The Shiatsu Centre
720 Bathurst Street, Suite 502
Toronto, Ontario
Canada M5S 2R4
Tel: 416-534-1140
Fax: 416-289-3627

Central Canada and Eastern United States
Heike Raschl (heike.raschl@gmail.com)
Tel: 416-516-6442 or 416-534-1140

Western Canada and Western United States
Cheryl Coull (cherylcoull@shaw.ca)
Tel: 250-388-0871
Meriel Cammell (shiatsu@saltspring.com)
Tel: 250-653-0055

Switzerland: Main European Office
Zita Sieber ZSI (info@zsi.ch)
Tel: 41-44-991-3142

Austria
Beatrix Simak (shiatsu@beatrixsimak.at)
Tel: 43-26-84-20021

Italy
Pietro Roat (pietro.roat@tiscali.it)
Tel: 39-0461-530244

Germany
Brigitte Pahl (shinso.shiatsu@alice-dsl.net)
Tel: 49 (0) 7252-536755
Marita Maier (mail@energieshiatsu.de)
Tel: 49 (0) 7202-941476
Matthias P. Wieck (info@ausbildung-shiatsu.de)
Tel: 49 (0) 391-662-8699

Australia-New Zealand
Estelita Pearce and Richard Malter (richardmalter@riseup.net)
Tel: 61-3-5348-3518
www.akoqi.com.au

Shin So Shiatsu International is associated with the following:

Shiatsu School of Canada
Enza Ierullo
547 College Street,
Toronto, Ontario
Canada M6G 1A9
Tel: 416-323-1818
admin@shiatsucanada.com

Sourcepoint Shiatsu Therapy Centre
Ted Thomas
3261 Heather St,
Vancouver, British Columbia,
Canada V5Z 3K4
Tel: 604-876-0042
ted_thomas@shaw.ca

Kiatsu School
(KIATSU Schule für Shiatsu)
Anneliese Haidinger
Seidengasse 32, 1070 Wien
Vienna, Austria
Tel: 43-1-522-2853
shiatsu@kiatsu.at

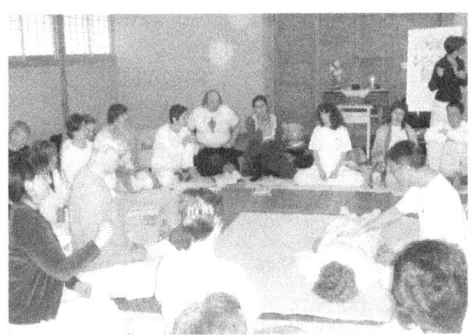
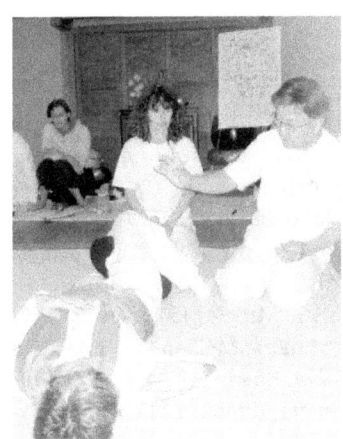

Ted Saito in Switzerland, April 2006.
Shin So Shiatsu organizer Zita Sieber, on Ted's right, is translating.

Suggested Reading

Shiatsu

Beresford-Cooke, Carola. 1996. *Shiatsu Theory and Practice.* Churchill-Livingstone, London.
Masunaga, Shizuto. 1987. *Meridian Exercises.* Japan Publications, Tokyo.
Masunaga, Shizuto. 1977. *Zen Shiatsu.* Japan Publications, Tokyo.
Masunaga, Shizuto. 1983. *Keiraku To Shiatsu.* Idono Nippon Sha, Japan.
Namikoshi, Toru. 1981. *The Complete Book of Shiatsu Therapy.* Japan Publications, Tokyo.

TCM and Meridian Theory

Fujita, Rokuro, M.D. 1980. *An Introduction to Meridianology.* Sogen Sha, Japan.
Kaneko, Ushinosuke. 1975. *Nippon Human Anatomy, Vols 1-3.* Nanzando Co, Ltd. Japan.
Low, Royston H. 1983. *The Secondary Vessels of Acupuncture.* Thorsons Publishing Group. England.
Maciocia, Giovanni. 1989. *The Fundamentals of Traditional Chinese Medicine.* Churchill-Livingstone, London.
Manaka Y, Itaya K, Birch S.1995. *Chasing the Dragon's Tail.* Paradigm Publications, Brookline, Massachusets.
Matsumoto, Kiiko with Birch, Stephen. 1986. *Extraordinary Vessels.* Paradigm Publications, Brookline, Massachusets.
Matsumoto, Kiiko with Birch, Stephen. 1988. *Hara Diagnosis: Reflections on the Sea.* Paradigm Publications, Brookline, Massachusets.
Shimi, Miki and Chase, Charles. 2001. *The Channel Divergences.* Blue Poppy Press, U.S.
Veith, Ilza. 1966. *The Yellow Emperor's Classic of Internal Medicine.* University of California Press, Berkely.

Working with Ki

Brennan, Barbara Ann. 1988. *Hands of Light.* Bantam Books, New York.
Cohen, Kenneth S. 1997. *The Way of Qigong.* Ballantine Books, New York.
Irie, Tadashi. 1982. *Keibetsu Keikin Kikei Ryoho.* Idono Nippon Sha, Japan.
Irie, Tadashi. 1990. Toyo *Igaku Genron.* Tadashi Irie, Japan.
Irie, Tadashi. 1991. *Kanpo Chiryo Genron.* Tadashi Irie, Japan.
Kushi, Michio. 1979. *The Book of Do-In.* Japan Publications, Tokyo.
Okudaira, Meikan. 1999. *Jaki Ron.* Idono Nippon Sha, Japan.
Tohei, Koichi. 1978. *Ki in Daily Life.* Ki No Kenkyukai, Tokyo.
Yokota, Kanpo. 1995. *Keiraku Ryuchu Kougi.* Idono Nippon Sha. Japan.
Yoshimoto, Hideo. 1996. *Ki Ketsu Sui Genro: Diagnosis and Treatment.* Hideo Yoshimoto, Japan.

Index

Please note:
Figures and Illustrations are listed on page xiii.
Where indicated, also refer to your *Reference Manual*.

A

abdominal diagnosis:
   by finger test 5, 6, 19;
   by palpation 5, 6, 19, 72, 73,74
abdominal diagnostic zones (Regular Meridians) 33,
   36, 73, (also see *Reference Manual*);
   comparison of Masunaga and Saito 34, 35;
   as energy circles 34; Saito charts 35;
   sensing 58
acupuncture points 22, 23 36;
   how to locate 107
Alarm Points 36
aluminum foil, confirming diagnoses 74
arm positions, in treatment of:
   Cosmic System 145;
   Divergent Meridians 121, 122, chart 121;
   Extra Meridians 103, 104, chart 103;
   Ocean System 137, 138,
   chart 137;
   Regular Meridians 78, chart 79;
   (also see *Reference Manual*)
arms, treatment of 42, 80

B

back diagnostic zones:
   chart 4, 40, (also see *Reference Manual*);
   Divergent Meridians 117;
   Masunaga's 37;
   Regular Meridians 33; 41;
   as meridian belt zones 37
Belt (Extra) Meridian 37, 86, 88, 80, 132, 133, 134;
   (also see *Reference Manual*)
belt zones for meridian systems:
   Divergent 38, 44, charts 121;
   Extra 38, 86, 94, charts 94;
   Regular 41,42,
   charts 38-42 (also see *Reference Manual*)
belt zones for Regular Meridians:
   Bladder 42, 43;
   Kidney 41, 42, 43;
   Large Intestine 41;
   Small Intestine 39;
   Triple Heater 41, (also see *Reference Manual*)
Bladder Meridian (Divergent) 112, 113,
   (also see *Reference Manual*)
Bladder Meridian (Regular) 29, 142,
   (also see *Reference Manual*);
   diagnostic zone, comparing Saito and Masunaga
   chart 34, 35;
   functions 42, 43, 134;
   overflow into Extra Meridian 90;
   treatment 81
Blood 133
blood, circulation 134
Bo Points 36
body alignment 6
brain, meridian functions 43
Brennan, Barbara Ann 149

C

cancer, treatment 72, 131
Chakra System 141, 147-151,
   (also see *Reference Manual*);
   diagnosis 151;
   Meridians 150;
   sensor 149;
   treatment 151
Chong Mai. See Penetrating Meridian
Conception Vessel 27, 43, 86, 87, 88, 90, 95;
   pathway 91, (also see *Reference Manual*)
Confirmation, of meridian diagnosis:
   Divergent 117, 119, 120;
   Extra 96;
   Ocean 136;
   Regular most kyo-jitsu 73-74,
   in third degree 75;
   Tai Kyoku 1 144;
   Tai Kyoku 2 145;
   (also see *Reference Manual*)
Confluent Points 86, **87**, 89;
   Extra Meridian treatment using 107,
   (also see *Reference Manual*)
Cosmic energy 37, 141
Cosmic System. See Tai Kyoku

Crossing Points 116;
   chart 123;
   Divergent Meridian treatment with 122-125,
   (also see *Reference Manual*)

D

Dai Mai. See Belt Meridian
diodes, in treatment 66, 67, 76
Divergent Meridians 4, 5, 36, 37, 43, 64, 98, **109-126**;
   arm positions 121;
   belt zones 38, 43, 44, 121;
   confirmation points 117;
   Crossing Points 123;
   diagnosis **116-117**;
   energy circles 120;
   hidden 120;
   leg positions 121;
   pathways 112, 114;
   sensor 117;
   treatment **118-126**;
   (also see *Reference Manual*)
Du Mai. See Governor Vessel

E

electromagnetic fields 53
emotional dysfunction 63
emotions, and meridian functions 134
energy circles 31-37, 64, 86;
   characteristics of 36;
   in Divergent Meridian treatment 120;
   in Extra Meridian diagnosis 92, 93, 96, 97, 99, 100,
   and treatment 100, 101;
   in structural imbalances 101;
   in Tai kyoku System 142;
   sensing 58;
   types of 36;
   (also see *Reference Manual*)
Extra Meridians 4, 5, 36, 37, 64, 99, **83-107**, 111, 118, 126, 131, 132, 133;
   belt zones 38, 86, 94,
   sensing 95;
   Confluent Points 87, 106;
   diagnosis **96-97**;
   energy circles 86, 92, 93, 101;
   honji treatment 98;
   hyoji treatment 98;
   pathways 89, 97;
   names 88;
   pelvic imbalances, treatment of 102;
   sensor 95;
   sound images 94;
   structural integrity, role in 90;
   TCM view of 86, 87;
   treatments **98-107**;
   (also see *Reference Manual*)
Extraordinary Vessels. See Extra Meridians 85
feet, and meridian functions 42

F

Finger Test Method 2, 3, 7, 20, 22, 33, 47, **49**, 53;
   instructions for 50;
   testing foods and supplements 52
   first-degree imbalance. See Regular Meridians
Fluids 133
Four Oceans 131, 132
Fujita, Rokuro Dr 22
frequency, of treatment 62

G

Gallbladder Meridian (Divergent) 112;
   (also see *Reference Manual*)
Gallbladder Meridian (Regular) 28, 43, 90, 91, 134, 142, (also see *Reference Manual*);
   comparing TCM and Saito 24;
   overflow into Extra Meridian 90
Governor Vessel 43, 86, 87, 88, 90;
   pathway 91;
   (also see *Reference Manual*)

H

hands, and meridian functions 42
Hara diagnosis. See abdominal diagnosis
hara diagnostic zones. See abdominal diagnostic zones
Hatsu-so-ketsu Points. See Confluent Points
Heart Constrictor Meridian (Divergent) 112;
   (also see *Reference Manual*)
Heart Constrictor Meridian (Regular) 43, 90, 132, 133, 135, 142, (also see *Reference Manual*);
   overflow into Extra Meridian 90
Heart Meridian (Divergent) 112, (also see *Reference Manual*)
   Heart Meridian (Regular) 90, 134, 142, (also see *Reference Manual*);
   overflow into Extra Meridian 90
Hei-myaku. See Regular Meridians, first-degree
hidden imbalance 138
hidden meridians 120
hidden symptoms 72
Hirata, Kurakichi 37, 43, 64, 99
Hirata Zones 37, 43, 44

honji treatment 63, 66, 76, 98, 126
Hua Shou 14
hyoji treatment 64, 66, 76, 98,126

I
Internal imbalances, diagnosing 65
Iokai Center 17
ion pumping. See IP cord treatment
IP cord treatment 64, 116;
    of Extra Meridians 106;
    of Divergent Meridians 122-125;
    (also see *Reference Manual*)
Irie, Tadashi Dr 2, 20, 44, **48**, 64, 99;
    Divergent Meridians 113

J
ja ki 36, **61-62**, 63, 64, 65, 66, 130, 134
ja ki, internal: removal of 137, 138, 145,
    in treatment of Divergent Meridians 121;
    Extra Meridians 104,105;
    Ocean system 138;
    organs 105;
    spine 105
ja ki, surface 7, 54: removal of **53**, 55, 64;
    in treatment room 67
Japan Shiatsu College 17
jistu. See kyo

K
Kato, Fusajiro Dr 17
Katsupaku Jin 14
Ketsu Kai Ocean Meridian 129, 130;
    related meridian 132;
    symptoms of imbalance 131
ki 1, **47-48**, **61-63**, 72, 88, 130;
    (also see *Reference Manual*)
Ki Kai Ocean Meridian 129, 130, 135, 138;
    related meridian 132;
    symptoms of imbalance 131;
    (also see *Reference Manual*)
Kidney Meridian (Divergent)112;
    (also see *Reference Manual*)
Kidney Meridian (Regular) 15, 28, 72, 73, 90, 132, 133,
    134, 135, 142, (also see *Reference Manual*);
    comparing Saito and Masunaga diagnostic zones 34, 35;
    comparing Saito and TCM pathway 23;
    overflow into Extra Meridian 90;
    symptoms of imbalance 16
Kidney Bo Point 28

Kishi, Tsutomu Dr 22
kyo 17, 71, 72, 76, 78, 98, 100, 126;
    diagnosis of 73, 74

L
Large Intestine Meridian (Divergent) 112, 114, 116,
    (also see *Reference Manual*)
Large Intestine Meridian (Regular) 15, 20, 27, 72, 73,
    90, 13, 134, 142;
    Saito pathway 21, (also see *Reference Manual*);
    overflow into Extra Meridian 90
Large Intestine abdominal diagnostic zone, Saito and
    Masunaga 34
leg positions, in treatment of (also see *Reference Manual*):
    Cosmic System 145;
    Divergent Meridians 121;
    Extra Meridians 103, 104;
    Ocean System 137, 138,
    chart 137;
    Regular Meridians 77, 78, 79
legs, treatment 42, 80
Liver Meridian (Divergent) 112, (also see *Reference Manual*)
Liver Meridian (Regular) 15, 41, 43, 73, 90, 91, 132,
    133, 134, 135, 142, (also see *Reference Manual*);
    overflow into Extra Meridian 90;
    stretch position 77
Lung Meridian (Divergent) 112, 114, 116, (also see
    Reference Manual)
Lung Meridian (Regular) 90, 142, (also see *Reference Manual*);
    overflow into Extra Meridian 90

M
magnets, in diagnosis 100
Manaka, Yoshio Dr. 66
Master Points, treatment 81
Masunaga, Shizuto 2, 5, **17**, 18, 33, 37, 41, 43, 47, 48, 61
Masunaga Shiatsu Meridian Chart 19, 28, 34
Masunaga back diagnostic chart 37, 41
Masunaga, Keiko 18
Mental problems, treatment of 104
meridian belt zones 31, 32, 33, **37-41**, 77, and organ functions 42-44
meridian charts:
    Masunaga Shiatsu Chart 17, 18, **19**, 20, 34;
    Saito Meridian Charts (see *Reference Manual*);
    TCM, discussion of 13, 14, 16, 17, 22, 23, 24, 25, 27, 28, 29
meridian stretch positions 33, 37, 41, 77, 78

meridian systems. See each meridian system,
    listed alphabetically
meridians. See each meridian,
    listed alphabetically by name
moxibustion 99
Mu Bun Sai 54; chart 104, (also see *Reference Manual*)
Mu Bun Sai ja ki removal 104, 122, 138, (also see
    Reference Manual)
Mu Points 36
muscle testing 49
Muscles, and meridian functions 134

N
Namikoshi, Tokujiro 2, 17
neck, treatment 81
nerves, and meridian function 43

O
Oceans System 4, **127-138**, (also see *Reference Manual*);
    arm positions 137,
    associated meridians 137,
    confirmation points 136;
    diagnosis 136;
    meridians 135;
    sensor 136;
    sound images 137;
    treatment **137-138**;
    zones, chart 137
Oda, Hajime Dr 52, 53, 130, 131
Okudaira, Meikan 62
organs, and meridian functions, 63, 126, 134
Oriental medicine 1, 13, 47, 126
O-ring test 49

P
Penetrating Meridian 27, 86, 88, 90, 103, 132, 133,
    134, (also see *Reference Manual*)
polarity 100, of fingers 76
prenatal ki 72, 78
press needles 76

R
Ratsu-ketsu Points 116, chart; Divergent Meridian
    treatment with 122-125;
    (also see *Reference Manual*)
Regular Meridians **11-30**, **69-82**, 4, 5, 7, 13, 14, 20, 37,
    78, 85, 86, 111, 112, 118, 126, 131, 132, 133, (also
    see *Reference Manual*);
    first degree 15, 26,
    abdominal chart 35, 71;
    second degree 15, 16, 26, 71,
    abdominal chart 35;
    diagnosis 74;
    third degree 15,16, 20, 26, 28, 29, 36, 71, 72, 88,
    111,
    abdominal chart 35;
    diagnosis 74;
    confirmation 73-75;
    treatment 76;
    arm positions for treatment 78-79;
    overlap with Divergent Meridians 115;
    characteristics of 22-25;
    diagnosis 71;
    pathways 25;
    sensors 56, 57
Ren Mai. See Conception Vessel

S
Sea of Blood. See Ketsu Kai
Sea of Marrow. See Zui Kai
Sea of Qi. See Ki Kai
Sea of Water and Grain. See Sui-Koku Kai
second-degree Regular Meridian imbalance.
    See Regular Meridians
sei ki 36, 62, 63, 64, 72, **61**
sensors, for finger test 49-50:
    Regular Meridians 56-57;
    Extra Meridians 95;
    Divergent Meridians 117;
    Oceans 136;
    Tai Kyoku 144, 145
    (also see *Reference Manual*)
Shi Kai (Four Oceans) 129, 131;
    related meridians 132;
    symptoms of imbalance 131
shiatsu treatment, basic 76;
    for Regular Meridians 80, 81;
    Extra Meridians 102-103, 105;
    Divergent Meridians 120, 122, 126;
    Ocean System 138;
    Tai Kyoku System 145
Shin So Shiatsu, advantages of 5;
    definition 3;
    post-graduate studies 8, 156
Sho-sei-byo. See Regular Meridians, third degree
Shu Points 118, 120, (also see *Reference Manual*)
Skin, and meridian functions 134
Small Intestine Meridian (Divergent)112, (also see
    Reference Manual)
Small Intestine Meridian (Regular) 23, 38, 90, 134,

142, (also see *Reference Manual*);
comparing TCM and Saito 25;
overflow into Extra Meridian 90
Small Intestine Meridian diagnostic zone 34
Sound images 52, 56, 65, (also see *Reference Manual*);
used in finding structural problems 66;
for clearing surface ja ki 44;
for Extra Meridians 94;
Oceans System 130
Spleen Bo Point 25
Spleen Meridian (Divergent) 112, (also see *Reference Manual*)
Spleen Meridian (Regular) 25, 90, 132, 133, 134, 138, 142, (also see *Reference Manual*);
overflow into Extra Meridian 90
Spleen Meridian (Ocean) 135, (also see *Reference Manual*)
Spleen Meridian diagnostic zone 37
Stomach Meridian (Divergent) 112, (also see *Reference Manual*)
Stomach Meridian (Regular) 15, 23, 72, 73, 90, 132, 133, 135, 142 (also see *Reference Manual*);
comparing TCM and Saito 25;
overflow into Extra Meridian 90
structural integrity, Extra Meridians role in 90
structural problems 6, 63, 98
diagnosis 65, 66;
treatment 101
Suehara, Masaaki 52
Sui-Koku Kai Ocean Meridian 129, 130, (also see *Reference Manual*);
related meridian 132;
symptoms of imbalance 131

T

Tai Kyoku System 4, 130, 135, 139-146, (also see *Reference Manual*);
confirmation points 144, 145;
diagnosis 144;
energy circles 142;
pathways 142, 143;
sensors 144, 145;
treatment 145;
treatment points 143
tanden 47, 49
TCM, view of: Regular Meridians 1, 13-29, 36, 42, 43, 62, 72, 80;
Extra Meridians 86, 87, 88, 89, 91, 106;
Divergent Meridians 112, 114, 115, 116;
Ocean Meridians 129, 130, 134

Third-degree Regular Meridian imbalance. See Regular Meridians
treatment responses 67, 126
Triple Heater Meridian (Divergent) 112, 134, (also see *Reference Manual*)
Triple Heater Meridian (Regular) 23, 43, 88, 90, 132, 134, 135, 142 (also see *Reference Manual*);
comparing Saito and Masunaga abdominal diagnostic zone 41;
overflow into Extra Meridian 90

V

vertebrae, locating 56 (also see *Reference Manual*)

Y

Yaki hari 63, 64; treatment with 99, 76, 118, 100;
treatment for structural imbalances 101, 102;
(also see *Reference Manual*)
Yang Connecting Meridian 86, 88, 90, 91, (also see *Reference Manual*)
Yang Heel Meridian 86, 88, 90, (also see *Reference Manual*)
Yang Qiao Mai. See Yang Heel Meridian
Yang Wei Mai. See Yang Connecting Meridian
Yin Connecting Meridian 86, 88, 90, 91, (also see *Reference Manual*)
Yin Heel Meridian 86, 88, 90, (also see *Reference Manual*)
Yin Qiao Mai. See Yin Heel Meridian
Yin Wei Mai. See Yin Connecting Meridian
Yin-Miyaku Kai Ocean Meridian 130;
related meridian 132;
(also see *Reference Manual*)
Yo-Miyaku Kai Ocean Meridian 130;
related meridian 132;
(also see *Reference Manual*)
Yoshimoto Chakra Sensor 149, (also see *Reference Manual*)
Yoshimoto, Hideo Dr 114, 49, 130, 131, 149
Yu Points 105

Z

Ze-do-byo. See Regular Meridians, second degree 15
Zen Shiatsu 5, 18, 34, 41, 49, 73
Zui Kai Ocean Meridian 129, 130;
related meridian 132;
symptoms of imbalance 131;
(also see *Reference Manual*)

www.ingramcontent.com/pod-product-compliance
Lightning Source LLC
Chambersburg PA
CBHW080806300426
44114CB00020B/2851